THE CARE ASSISTANT'S GUIDE

to working with

PEOPLE WITH DEMENTIA

Edited by Sue Benson

PUBLISHED BY
Journal of Dementia Care

4TH EDITION

This fourth edition published in 2002 by
Hawker Publications Ltd
Culvert House
Culvert Road
London SW11 5DH
Tel: 020 7720 2108

1st Edition published in 1991. Reprinted 1992.
2nd Edition published in 1994. 3rd Edition published in 1998.

British Library Cataloguing in Publication Data
A catalogue record for this book is available from the British Library

ISBN 1 874790 70 1

Designed by
Richard Souper and Sue Lishman

Phototypeset by
Hawker Publications

Printed and bound in Great Britain by
BR Hubbard, Dronfield, Sheffield

Other titles in this series:
Handbook for Care Assistants – A Practical Guide to Caring for Elderly People
Sixth Edition 2003. ISBN 1 874790 69 8
A Practical Guide to Working with People With Learning Disabilities
Second Edition 1994. ISBN 1 874790 12 4

Other publications from Hawker Publications include:
Dementia Topics for the Millennium and Beyond. Edited by Sue Benson (2002).
ISBN 1 874790 64 7.
Care Homes and Dementia. Edited by Sue Benson (2001). ISBN 1 874790 57 4.
Care to Communicate. By Jennie Powell (2000). ISBN 1 874790 48 5.
Person-Centred Care. Edited by Sue Benson (2000). ISBN 1 874790 54 X.
Improving Dementia Care: a resource for training and professional development.
By Buz Loveday, Tom Kitwood and Brenda Bowe (1998). ISBN 1 874790 38 8.
Design for Dementia. Edited by Stephen Judd, Mary Marshall and Peter Phippen
(1997). ISBN 1 874790 35 3.

Hawker Publications also publishes The Journal of Dementia Care,
a bi-monthly journal for all practitioners caring for people with dementia.
For further information write to the editor at the address above or email
sue@hawkerpubs.demon.co.uk
See also our website: www.dementia.careinfo.org

Contents

Contributors

June Andrews RMN RGN MA is director of nursing, at Forth Valley Acute Hospital NHS Trust. Her experience has been in nursing elderly and elderly mentally ill people.

Carole Archibald BA RGN HV is senior fieldworker at the Dementia Services Development Centre, University of Stirling. She has worked in the field of dementia care for fifteen years. Her interests include activities for people with dementia, respite care, specialist dementia units and sexuality.

Michael Broughton RGN RMN DipN is dementia services manager for Methodist Homes, a major provider of Christian-based care with three specialist homes for people with dementia. He previously worked as a manager for Ashbourne Homes.

Karen Bryan PhD BSc MCSLT is a lecturer in acquired communication disorders at the National Hospitals College of Speech Sciences. She is currently involved in developing a communication training programme for care assistants.

Cathy Chatten BA RGN RMN MN PGCE wrote this chapter while clinical effectiveness co-ordinator for Cardiff Community Healthcare NHS Trust. She has extensive clinical experience in dementia care, and facilitates a training course for care workers. She has also been a lecturer in Care of the Elderly and Mental Health for the Department of Nursing Studies, University of Wales College of Medicine, where she is a research fellow.

Joan Costello RGN wrote this chapter while home manager of Westbury, Methodist Homes' specialist care home for people with dementia.

Valerie Good is manager of mental health services for older people for East Sussex County Healthcare NHS Trust. Formerly a psychiatric social worker, she has worked with older people for the last 20 years, in a multi-disciplinary team setting, managing a range of services including resource centres, and in the strategic development of a range of innovative services. She is particularly interested in the development of new forms of residential provision for people with dementia.

Brenda Hooper MA. Until her recent death, Brenda worked as a specialist consultant, author and trainer in dementia care. She was previously a residential home manager, and training adviser for the Centre for Policy on Ageing.

Alison Johnson MA is an independent consultant and writer in dementia care. Formerly she was secretary to Methodist Homes, with responsibility for research, information and strategic planning. She visited Australia in early 1997 as a Winston Churchill Fellow, looking at design and care practices for people with dementia.

Michael Maltby BSc DipClinPsych AFBPS CPsychol is a clinical psychologist with Tunbridge Wells Health Authority. He specialises in work with older people and carers, including staff training and consultancy.

Jim Marr is director of care and quality for Barchester Healthcare. For many years he has been involved in promoting the specialist care of older people, particularly those with dementia, working on national policy formation, education and management issues.

Jane Maxim PhD MA DipCST MCSLT is a senior lecturer at the National Hospitals College of Speech Sciences. She is a speech therapist whose research area is language change in dementia, and she works with elderly stroke patients.

Tracy Packer RGN is nurse consultant in dementia care (acute services) for North Bristol NHS Trust, Bristol. She is involved in training and developing strategies with staff to improve the wellbeing of people with dementia. She previously worked in the acute elderly care unit at St Mary's Hospital, Paddington, where she was appointed senior staff nurse and then acting ward manager.

Tessa Perrin wrote this chapter while working as senior practitioner occupational therapist for Essex Social Services. She recently completed a period of secondment to the Bradford Dementia Group, where she investigated the role and value of occupation in the treatment of persons with severe dementia.

Lynne Phair MA RGN RMN BSc (Hons) Nursing DPNS is nursing and care manager at RSAS Agecare. She has specialised in the care of older people with mental health problems and worked in acute assessment, the community, joint health and social services care settings in the NHS before moving into the voluntary sector. She has a special interest in the quality of care, and a desire to achieve equality in the quality of care for people with dementia.

Maria Scurfield is clinical nurse manager at Monkwearmouth Hospital, Sunderland. She has extensive clinical experience in the dementia care field, has worked with Bradford Dementia Group and for the Royal College of Nursing's special interest group, now called the *RCN Mental Health and Older People Forum.*

Margaret Anne Tibbs, currently a freelance writer and trainer on dementia care, previously worked as senior social worker with the Pathfinder Team, closely involved with dementia-specific residential homes and day care facilities. She has specialised in dementia care since 1989, having first become interested in this field in South Africa where she worked in a private residential home after graduating in social work.

Michael Wafer BSc RGN RNMH wrote this chapter while working as senior nurse (quality assurance) at the Nursing Development Unit for Older People, Tameside Hospital, Lancashire.

Daphne Wallace recently retired as consultant in old age psychiatry at High Royds Hospital, Menston, West Yorkshire. She is also a Trustee of the Alzheimer's Society.

Bob Woods is professor of clinical psychology of older people at the University of Wales, Bangor, where he combines research and teaching with clinical work with older people and their families. He previously worked for many years in London, and has written and taught extensively on dementia care and related topics.

Photographs are by Sue Benson unless otherwise attributed. Many thanks to all residents and staff involved: AgeCare – pages 8, 14, 154; Westminster Health Care – pages 28, 62; Adamwood, Edinburgh – page 110; Darnall Dementia Group, Sheffield – 39, 161. Grange Day Unit, Sunderland – page 90.

Introduction

The world of dementia care has undergone a cultural revolution in recent years. In this new culture, where each person is valued and cared for as a unique individual, the role of the care assistant takes up a central position. We know now that there is a great deal that all care staff can do to maximise the wellbeing of people with dementia, despite the growing disabilities the disease brings.

With this new status and role of the care assistant comes a need for training. This book provides the underpinning knowledge and practical skills care assistants need for their day-to-day work in this specialist field. Its chapters, all written by authors whose breadth of knowledge is grounded in sound practical experience in dementia care, form a reliable guide to help staff understand and respond to the opportunities and challenges they encounter. Designed for all care assistants working with people with dementia in all long-term care settings – residential and nursing homes, and hospitals – it is relevant to day care settings too. It provides an essential framework for NVQ qualifications in care (levels 2 and 3).

In this new edition we have retained the individual voices of our authors, and their wisdom distilled from years of experience. One theme runs through all the chapters: that each person with dementia deserves to be treated with respect and careful attention to their needs, preferences and desires – especially those who are least able to make their wants known. This is the message we hope sounds loud and clear from the pages of this book. It is also the reason why you will not find terms like person-centred care, independence, dignity, individuality, self-esteem, choice, opportunity or equality in the index: these themes are central to every chapter.

We hope this new edition will continue to meet the needs of both care assistants and those responsible for their training, as a practical teaching resource to further the aim we all share, of high quality, truly person-centred care.

Sue Benson
Editor, *Journal of Dementia Care*

Foreword

By Tom Kitwood, Leader, Bradford Dementia Group,
University of Bradford

This book is a treasure-store of insight, information and guidance for the care of older people who have dementia. It brings together the wisdom and vision of twenty different contributors who have been deeply committed to the improvement of care practice. Together they represent all the main disciplines involved in this field - nursing, social work, occupational therapy, psychology and psychiatry - each presenting the fruit of their experience in a very readable way. As such the book is a unique production, and one which will, I am sure, prove to be of great value to all practitioners.

Although a variety of viewpoints is presented here, there is a common theme running through every contribution. It is that men and women who have dementia are, first and foremost, persons, and deserve to be treated as such. We can do a great deal to enable them to continue to be persons, even in the face of their disability and the accompanying emotional problems. In many ways the old adage "Do as you would be done by" is the message, and we can apply a simple test in assessing the quality of any care environment: "How would I myself like to be here, if I were to develop dementia?"

Good care involves having a stock of detailed knowledge, and skills that are specific to caring for older people whose mental powers are failing. We need to know how to recognise depression, for example, and understand its relationship to dementia. We need to understand the principles and practice of good communication. We need a sound grasp of issues related to nutrition, general health and the management of pain. We need to be able to form good relationships with family members, and have empathy with their experience. In a multicultural society, it is vital to know something about the background and religion of each of the main minority ethnic groups. All this, and much more, will be found here.

Over the last few years many advances have been made in the care of people with dementia. At last this is being recognized as a form of work that involves great skill and insight, and a very highly developed range of human qualities. It is important, then, that all who are involved in this field, at whatever level of seniority, have the chance to keep up to date with new developments in practice. This book will enable the reader to do this. Everyone who succeeds in following through what is written here will have a resource which will help them to become an excellent practitioner of care; and I am sure they will find that their effort and commitment are richly rewarded.

Tom Kitwood, 1998

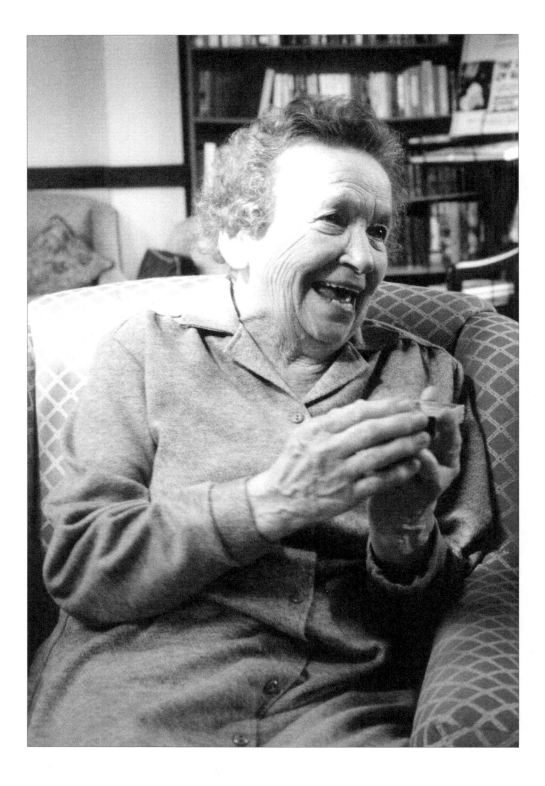

CHAPTER 1

Discovering the person

Margaret Anne Tibbs

• Look for the person first and the dementia second
• We need to know as much about the person as possible • Individualised activities
• Communicate in a way which makes sense to them • Life story work
and reminiscence • Spirituality and religion

When we are caring for a person with dementia it is essential that we always remember the following basic truth:

We look for the person first and the dementia second.

This may sound like common sense. But it can be very easy to fall into the trap of concentrating on the illness and the problems it brings, for the person and for those of us who care for them. In doing this we can lose sight of the person who was there before the illness developed and who, we believe, is still there.

Many assessments continue to concentrate on the things the person cannot do, to the point where all the things which they can do are forgotten.

It is, of course, necessary to know which tasks the person can no longer perform for themself in order to create a proper care plan and minimise risk. But we want to help the person to feel as good about themself as possible. In order to do this we need to emphasise the things a person can still do and concentrate on them. So we need to know as much about the person as possible.

Why do we need to know?

• We can easily make misjudgements about people through ignorance

• We can misunderstand a person's words and actions

• We can give serious offence

• We can make people irritated, frightened, threatened or angry by our own actions which are intended to help them.

What sort of things do we need to know?

We need to know who they are
This sounds so obvious that it does not need saying. But I do not mean their name, their age, where they used to live, or how old they are.

I mean the things which are important about them. These are the same things which are important about yourself. The things which you would want anyone to understand about you if you were in a situation where you depended upon other people for your comfort and happiness.

We need to know what kind of a person they were before they became disabled by dementia.

What was their personality?

• Were they passive, happy to fit in with other people or did they take the lead ?
• Were they generally even tempered or did they easily become irritated?
• Were they calm and confident or prone to anxiety or depression?
• What sort of things did they like to do?
• Were they physically very active, enjoying sports or long walks?
• Were they an animal lover or were they afraid of dogs?
• What were their hobbies? Did they like painting, reading, sewing, knitting or were they a bit of a couch potato?
• What was their attitude to taking medication? Were they the kind of person who mistrusts tablets? Or would they have asked for "a pill for every ill"?

More important possibly than their leisure interests is what they did as an occupation. The oldest female residents were probably wives and mothers. In other words they spent their adult life caring for other people. They were also probably housewives and would have been always busy with household tasks.

With the men it is important to know what their job was. Did they work with their hands or did they have an office job?. Were they in charge of other people or were they used to being told what to do?

We tend to assume that none of the women who were born in the first two decades of the twentieth century had a career. We often assume that they were fully occupied as wives and/or mothers. While this was true in general, many women had jobs or careers which may well have been important to them. It is important to check this.

For the people who are in residential care at present it is important to know what happened to them in the Second World War. This was a very important and significant time for most of the men and

Joan was seen as "difficult" at the day hospital because she did not want to join in with group activities. When she talked about the amazing things she had done it was assumed that she was rambling because the nurses found it hard to see beyond the frail body and the confused mind.

We should never just dismiss the stories someone tells of their life. This little old lady had been a heroine in the last war, working as a British agent with the French resistance. It was not surprising that someone who must have been extremely self reliant, independent, not to mention courageous, should have found it hard to settle down in a group to colour in Christmas cards. What she did like to do was to talk on a one to one basis with the staff about herself.

many of the women who lived through it. Any man born before 1920 would have been involved in some way. For those men who served in the armed forces, the experience would have changed their lives. Apart from the traumatic experience of combat and multiple losses as friends and comrades were killed, it was also the first time that many men had been away from home.

You should be particularly aware of the devastating effects that being a prisoner of war had on people. This seems to be especially true of men who were taken prisoner in the Far East. It appears that many men have never talked about the dark side of their war experiences. When dementia develops they are forced to relive memories which have been long buried. Should you ever come across a victim of the Holocaust who has dementia, they may well need specialist counselling. The same is true of immigrants from countries in the former Soviet

Union who have settled in the UK.

Remember that civilians throughout the UK were bombed. They lived through a time of great hardship when every basic thing that is normally used in the home was rationed. It was often very cold. These conditions of hardship lasted for several years after the war had ended. The winter of 1947 was one of the coldest ever recorded and coal, the only form of heating then, was rationed.

However, for many women, the war provided an opportunity to work, to earn money and to gain independence for the first time. The country needed them to do so because all the men were away fighting (apart from those in Reserved Occupations whose skills were vitally needed at home). They also had to take all the decisions about the home and children which the men would have made before.

Early in the war, children from the big cities were evacuated to keep them safe from the bombing. These children are now coming up to the age where some will need residential care. Evacuees were sent away from home to live in the country. A massive operation was organised and children were dispatched from their schools, each with a luggage label with their name and address on it and clutching their gas masks in cardboard boxes. Some children, after the initial terror of separation, had good experiences with loving families. For others the experience was traumatic: they were not wanted and not cared for. Children from the same family might be separated because they could not be offered accommodation together, which added to the feelings of loss, fear and rejection.

But many people look back on this period with nostalgia. This is because everybody was working together – quite literally – for survival. This generated good feelings of community, sharing, mutual support and a feeling of solidarity.

So remember, people's experiences of the war were very different. Because those six years between 1939 and 1945 made such a profound impression on everybody, they can be very useful as a reminiscence tool (see chapter 4). But you must find out, to the best of your ability, what the experience was like for each individual in your care.

What are their values and beliefs? We all have strong beliefs about something – politics, patriotism as well as religion. Again it is easy to assume that because a person is of a particular age they will hold a particular view about something.

What ethnic and cultural background do they come from? It is essential to get this right. (The subject will be covered in chapter 2.)

Communication

In order for a person with dementia to feel as good about themselves as possible, **we should communicate with them in a way which makes sense to them.**

This may take more time in the beginning, but you will help the person as well as saving time in the end, by doing the following things:

- **Find out how they like to be addressed.** Do not assume that calling a person by their first name is a sign of friendship. To some older people it is seen as patronising, disrespectful or downright rude. They may not be able to tell you how they feel in words, but they certainly will in their actions.

- **Try to enter the world in which they find themselves.** Because their short term memory is likely to be impaired by now, they may be "living" in a place which is unfamiliar to you. A person in their mid eighties who has lost sixty years' worth of memories is likely to be talking about and reacting to things which happened in another time, another place. They are not simply talking nonsense.

• **Try to share their world as much as you can.** Ask them to tell you about the past. You can often learn a great deal from them about the history of the place where your care home is situated, if they have lived there all their lives.

How do we find out who the person is?

• By asking the person to tell you.

• By asking family and friends about them. If they have nobody left who knew them in earlier times, we must find out as much as we can by reading or talking to other people who are sources of local knowledge.

At the point of introduction to the residential unit there should be a partnership between the community staff, social workers and nurses, the person with dementia and their family so that as much information as possible may be passed on to the home.

This does not mean only the obvious things like medication and diet and the name of the main carer. All this information should be put on to the form which is completed when they first come in.

What I mean is **much** more detailed information about their former lifestyle. For example:

• What time do they normally get up, and when do they like to go to bed?

• How do they usually like to spend their days?

• Are they used to going out on their own? If the answer is yes the next question must be, are they safe?

This will have to be tested by the staff initially. If a person's road sense is still intact they can obviously go out with others. Once they have accepted that they now live with you and they have been

> Tom, who had been a school caretaker, appeared to achieve a sense of satisfaction from washing down the minibus at the residential home where he lives.
>
> Miss Eleanor Jeeves, who was head of the language department at a local public school, enjoys talking French to a nurse from Mauritius in the nursing home. Her French is, apparently, of a much higher standard than his own.

tested to see whether they can find their way back to you, they may be allowed to take themselves in and out on their own. There may well be a difference between the perception of the relatives who see the need for safety as all important, and care staff who feel that the person is entitled to some independence (see chapter 5).

Remember: there is no such thing as a risk free environment for any of us, though we often attempt to create such an environment for a person with dementia. The problem is that by doing so we often seriously damage the person's quality of life.

We need to know if there are elements of their former occupation which they can still perform. Women who have been housewives may enjoy helping to wash up or dust furniture. Mothers may enjoy caring for other residents who are more frail than they are. These things will help them to feel better about themselves. In the box above are examples of people who are still able to feel valuable because they are doing something which was valued when they were younger.

We should find out if the person had a hobby which, with help, could be started again. This may happen even if, living alone at home, they have apparently lost interest in it.

What about personal space? Are they

Fred, who was aged 80, was seen to remove all tablets from his mouth after they had been given to him, and go to elaborate lengths to hide them, burying them in plant pots or hiding them in his clothing. He also reacted with extreme fear when a staff member approached him with a request to do something, such as move to the dining room.

It was only when his wife mentioned in passing that he had been a Japanese prisoner of war, that the staff understood what was happening. He obviously knew that he was no longer at home and misinterpreted the situation so that he thought he was back in the POW camp. He obviously was not going to accept pills which he thought might harm him, but dared not refuse outright. Similarly he overreacted to staff requests which he interpreted as orders from the people in charge, who had to be hostile.

After this the staff adopted an extremely gentle approach to him. His medication was changed to a liquid form which, fortunately, he did not perceive as threatening. He gradually settled down in the home.

the sort of person who needs a lot of personal space and would prefer to spend a lot of time in their own room?

Or are they sociable, always seeking out the company of others? They may have been intensely lonely living on their own at home, and this seeking out the company of other people may have been misinterpreted. They may have been labelled as a nuisance, always pestering other people, by the warden of the sheltered flats. People like this may blossom very quickly in the environment of a residential home where there are always people around.

Others, however, may find it very stressful to be constantly in the company of other people. Constant noise and activity may be difficult for them to tolerate.

Life story records

A very good way to build up a picture of a person's life is to make a record in picture form in a photo album, or on audio tape. With the help of the person's family and friends you can obtain photos of people and places which were important to the person in your care. These will need to be labelled of course with names and dates. Pictures of topics which have been significant can also be included. Compiling a book like this can be an interesting and helpful project for the person's family. They may well be feeling guilty as well as sad that the person can no longer live at home.

The same can be done with music – using tracks of records – if the person enjoys music.

Once completed, these books or tapes can be kept somewhere safe in the home and used by care staff as well as the family when they visit, as a means of encouraging them to talk about their past lives. This reminiscence work (see chapter 4) is a valuable tool. Prompts such as their own life story records, pictures or objects from the past, are keys which you can use to open the door for them – a door into happier times before they became disabled by dementia. It enables them to escape from their present world, where they cannot remember and as a result are often afraid and bewildered, into a world where they are sure of themselves, where they have interesting things to tell you – *which you don't know.*

This puts them, for once, in a position of knowing more than you do. It makes them feel good about themselves. Those feelings of confidence and happiness will

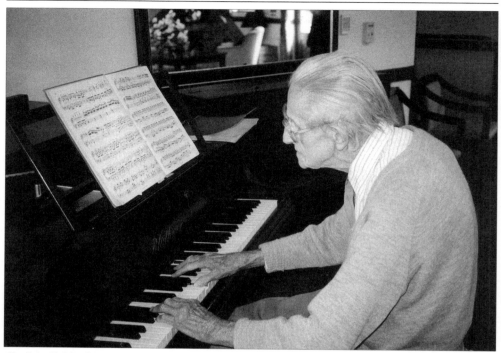

Each individual is unique with their own skills, tastes, and social and educational background.

persist for some time after they have forgotten your reminiscence session, and will add greatly to their quality of life.

You may be surprised by the knowledge which the person with dementia has about the family. Very old people are a vital source of family history and may remember things which other family members do not. Every family has a family history, and this is really important to each generation. With help, the person with dementia may be able to share interesting stories with the rest of their family.

Memories of young adulthood seem to be the most vivid. The time when people first went to work, fell in love, had babies, moved away from home. For many men over 80 the war years seem to have been the most significant of their lives, which is hardly surprising. Tread carefully however, because the memories may be very painful ones.

Often crucial pieces of information

which provide the key to understanding a person's behaviour are not known by staff when they come into the home

Once you have learned as much as possible about the person with dementia you will be able to develop customised reminiscence activities for them (as well as other activities – see chapter 8).

Reminiscence is a very valuable tool for staff who work with people with dementia. Some reminiscence can be happily shared by a group of people of roughly the same age and social group who have lived in the same geographical area. We can safely assume that they will have certain memories in common.

But in order to be effective in building up the self esteem of a person, rather than just a reasonably pleasant way of passing an hour together, the careworker must have a detailed knowledge of the person in their care.

The same applies to activities. Watching

videos of the royal family or community singing is better than sitting in a chair doing nothing. But if activities are to be valuable and productive they must be customised to meet the needs of each individual person in the home (see chapters 5 and 8).

All people are different

This is something we should remember all the time.

Not everyone enjoys group activities such as community singing, ball games etc. Many people have never been "joiners". They may have run a mile from joining a club. There is no reason why, because they have dementia, they should be expected to do so now.

As well as coming from different ethnic backgrounds people come from different social backgrounds.

It makes life easier for the staff if they assume that all people enjoy doing the same things when they are living in a communal setting. People in residential homes who are physically frail can make it very clear what they do or do not want to do. People with dementia cannot tell us.

We must learn to celebrate our differences and not try to make everyone do the same thing. Because it is quicker and easier to organise all the residents into doing the same activity, or eating the same thing at the same time, or going to bed at the same time, we fail to offer people a choice. We are all entitled to a choice about the way we live, even if we are living in a community with other people.

> Some people like Radio 2, others like Classic FM. We don't all like the same TV programmes. The list of possible differences between people is endless.

> Some men, who are always in a minority in residential homes because women live longer, enjoy spending most of their time with women (staff as well as residents). Other men hate it. They really long for the company of other men. Some women are not used to being in the company of men at all.

It takes time to offer choice and allow people to be different. but if we do make the time we will find that people are happier in themselves. They will feel valued for who they are, even as the illnesses progress. This in turn will make management of the home smoother and easier.

People may not be able to communicate their good feelings in words but the result will be shown in their behaviour. Actions speak louder than words.

We now believe that people with dementia do communicate in all sorts of ways, with the people who look after them. We have to learn this communication – rather like learning a foreign language. (See also chapters 3, 4 and 5.)

Sarah

Sarah had recently arrived at the home. She was constantly trying to leave the building. She hovered near the front door. She had been found trying to go out through the fire exit. When staff members asked her where she was going, she said she had to get back home because her mother was waiting for her. She became tearful and was clearly upset.

What was she trying to tell the staff?
Look at what she was doing. Remember: actions speak louder than words. We only try to leave a place if we don't want to be there – if we are unhappy. She said she had to go back to her mother. There is

no way her mother could still be alive. But what was she trying to communicate?

What does "mother" stand for?

It stands for feeling safe, feeling loved, feeling protected. All the things she was not feeling. She was telling the staff that she felt vulnerable, helpless, as frightened as a child and in desperate need of comfort.

What else was she doing?

Her tears and her pacing up and down showed that she was distressed, restless and frightened, wanting to get away from a situation of tension. How often have you felt like that?

She had no idea where she was or how she got there. She had no idea who the staff were and was not absolutely sure that they could be trusted.

She was desperate for reassurance and comfort. She told the staff all this without being able to say so in words. They had to tune in to her language to open up communication with her, and so help

Expressing their feelings

People with dementia often use the language of pictures. Pictures which are very vivid and powerful. The actual words of the sentences they are saying may not make sense – they could not possibly be describing an event which happened a few minutes ago in the home – but the pictures which they conjure up will tell you a lot about the way they feel.

Or they may use a lot of words in what seems to be a nonsensical way, but if you pick out odd phrases, half sentences from all the jumble of words, you can piece together a statement which makes sense. Often they are expressing deeply felt emotions, to do with loss and loneliness.

All this shows how vitally important it is to get to know the person with dementia

really well. They can no longer communicate effectively in your language, so you have to take the initiative and learn their language.

Spirituality and religion

These areas are of vital importance to many of us. They survive at a very deep level: spiritual and religious beliefs can be reached even when dementia is advanced, and they can become a lifeline – a strong rope to hang on to. It is extremely important to find out what things are important to the people in our care. This will probably become clear over a period of time. Because religious teaching has often been acquired by learning by heart, things like hymns, religious songs and passages can be recalled even at an advanced stage of the dementing illness.

Hymns, psalms, bible passages and other sacred writings can be recalled with help even though the short term memory is seriously impaired. They can be a great comfort.

On the other hand it may happen that a person who was religious all their life may turn against it. Again we need to follow the lead of the person, and understand what they are trying to communicate to us.

Remember, spirituality does not have to have anything to do with religion. People may have deeply held feelings about nature, music, poetry. All these can be used to reach the person inside where they still live, beyond the destruction of their brain cells.

We have returned to the same theme. Listen to what people do, not just what they say.

It is important for us to remember that all human beings are unique. The fact that the people in our care are disabled by dementia means that they share certain symptoms which cause unusual kinds of behaviour. These symptoms are not the most important thing about them. We should not focus on the things they cannot do. The traditional way of looking after people with dementia was to concentrate on their problems and the difficulties which their problems caused for other people.

We should concentrate instead on the personality – the qualities and skills (past and present) which have made them the unique person they are.

In order to do this we have to find a way to allow them to be themselves, while offering them the care and support they need. This is not an easy task. We may try and we may fail. When we fail we have to try again – and again.

It is only by treating each person with dementia as a unique and valuable human being that we will be able to create an environment in which they will be able to find the highest quality of life which is possible for them.

Points to remember

1. We look for the person first and the dementia second.

2. In order to be able to find the person we need to know as much about them as possible.

3. We have to learn to communicate with the person with dementia in a way that makes sense to them. This may be time-consuming at the beginning but will save time in the end, because the person will trust you and cooperate with you.

4. We find out who the person is by asking them, and taking time to listen. We also find out as much as we can from family and friends.

5. The management of risk is vitally important. We have to achieve a balancing act between risk and quality of life. Remember, there is no such thing as a risk-free environment for any of us. Life story records are valuable as a means of building up a picture of a person's whole life before they came to live in your home.

6. Reminiscence work is best carried out on an individual basis, using the life story records. It helps the person feel better about themself. But it should always be done sensitively. Make sure you have "done your homework" to prepare for a session.

7. Always remember that all people are different. Activities which some people enjoy, others may dislike. People with dementia often cannot tell you in words that they are not enjoying something. Be sensitive to differences in gender and ethnic groups in particular.

8. Although it seems to save time and make life easier for the staff to treat everyone the same, this is not so. People are different and should be given as much choice as possible. They will be much happier if you do this.

9. Spiritual and religious ideas and traditions can often be a lifeline for people with dementia. They can act as a strong link with the past, and with what is most important to the person. Try to find out about them, and use them.

CHAPTER 2

Special needs of minority ethnic groups

Margaret Anne Tibbs

- *Learning about someone's racial, cultural and religious background is a vital part of person-centred care* • *Different languages and religions*
- *Body language and its different meanings*

We have seen in the last chapter how important it is to find out as much as we possibly can about the person with dementia in order to help them find the best quality of life which is possible for them. This is hard enough if the person comes from the same cultural background as we do.

If the person comes from a different ethnic and/or religious group from us, it becomes even harder. It is, however, even more important for us to find out all about their culture, their customs, tastes and preferences, and the things that are most important to them.

In the UK we find people from a variety of different cultures. Even within those whose families have lived here for many centuries we find different groups. We have Scots, Welsh and Irish people, each with their own distinctive history and national identity. We have the difference between north and south of England.

Long ago the original inhabitants of the islands that make up the UK were invaded by warriors from many different countries – the Normans from France, the Vikings from Scandanavia, and the Romans from Italy, They came as invaders and remained as settlers.

Since those very early days many immigrants have also settled here – many came fleeing from persecution. Over time they have become absorbed into the host population. But these groups still hold on to their own national customs, beliefs and religions, which are many and varied.

In the 1950s and 1960s large numbers of people from the Caribbean and the Indian subcontinent were recruited to work here. Those groups are of significant size, and first settlers have now reached the age where they may be needing residential or nursing care.

There are, of course, sizeable populations in different parts of the UK from other European countries. They are also reaching the age group with which we are concerned. There are groups from the countries in the former Soviet Union, Italy, Hong Kong, Vietnam etc. In fact there are groups from many countries who have settled here and made this country their home.

There are two important and different ways to classify people from minority ethnic groups:
- Language
- Religion.

Language

Language is obviously very important, as people with dementia who learned English as a second language will probably have forgotten most or all of it. Because of impaired short term memory, they often revert to speaking entirely in their mother tongue (the language in which they first learned to speak).

Interpreters are important, but we need people who can understand the special needs of people with dementia as well as those who can speak the language.

Do not rely on relatives for interpretation. They will have their own agenda. They will often tell you that the language does not matter because the person is talking nonsense anyway. You will realise, with your specialised knowledge of dementia, that this is not always true.

If it is at all possible, find someone who speaks the person's language. The manager of the home should be aware of what the common languages in your locality are, and have a list of accredited interpreters available.

A complete list of languages other than English spoken in the UK is too long to give here, but common languages are:

Bengali, Hindi or *Urdu* – people from Bangladesh
Cantonese or *Hakka* – people from Hong Kong
Urdu or *Punjabi* – people from Pakistan
Punjabi or *Hindi* – Sikhs and Hindus from Punjab
Gujarati or *Hindi* – Indians from Gujarat.

Body language is also extremely important. It may have quite different meanings for people from different cultures.

The personal space and physical contact people find comfortable differs in different cultures. A friendly hug from a white European may be interpreted by a Chinese person as over familiarity. A noisy conversation between people from a Caribbean or Mediterranean country may be interpreted as an argument or a threat when they are just being emphatic.

African men may hold hands with each other. If white British men did so we might assume they were gay. An Asian woman does not make eye contact. This is interpreted by white Europeans as shifty. It is assumed that she is being evasive. In fact she is showing respect. The examples could be endless and there are many possibilities for misunderstanding.

It is very important to learn through observation, asking someone from the same cultural group, or reading about the subject, what the important differences in body language are if the person comes from an ethnic group which is different from your own.

Religions

The great world religions are all represented in the UK: Buddhism, Hinduism, Islam, Judaism, Sikhism, and of course, Christianity.

All have different customs about birth, marriage, sickness and death. Attitudes towards mental illness and dementia will be very different as well. We will look very briefly at these religions.

Buddhism

Buddhism is based on the teachings of Gautama the Buddha who was born about 563 BC in North India.

Buddhists seek enlightenment and they attempt to do this through living a life based on meditation and simplicity of lifestyle and self control. They believe the enlightenment which Buddha found can be achieved through following the Eightfold Path, and that the essence of

Buddha is within each person. Buddhists believe in reincarnation.

Worship

Buddhists worship in a centre called a Vihara. It contains a shrine and usually has accommodation facilities for the community of teachers or monks. These monks are easy to recognise because they wear orange coloured robes and have shaven heads. Most Buddhists will make a shrine in their own home. This consists of a small table with a statue or picture of Buddha with flowers, candles and incense around it.

Although Buddhism began in India it is spreading in the West; there are around 130,000 practising Buddhists in the UK.

Diet

Buddhists are normally vegetarians, or try to be, because the Buddha's teaching about non-violence included all living creatures. Meals will vary according to where the person lived.

Dress

Nothing specific. People wear the usual dress of the country in which they live.

Attitudes to illness and medical/care staff

Because helping people is fundamental to Buddhist ideas, they will always respect doctors, nurses and care staff.

Death and dying

Buddhists believe in life after death (reincarnation). They believe that their actions in this life will have consequences in future lives as well as this one. If it is possible arrangements should be made for a Buddhist teacher or monk to be present when a Buddhist is dying. You will need to have the name of a person to contact anyway. The necessary prayers usually take an hour or so. They do not have to be said in the presence of the deceased.

The dead person will be cremated.

Hinduism

Hinduism is actually a collection of different forms of Indian beliefs rather than a single religion. It did not have a specific founder like the other world religions. There are probably about 400,000 Hindus in the UK.

Hindus believe in a supreme spirit of all creation. This spirit created all the hundreds of Hindu gods. The three most important are:

Brahma - Creator of Life
Vishnu - Preserver of Life
Siva - Destroyer of Life.

The many gods and goddesses are seen as different aspects of the same God.

Hindus believe that the soul must be cleansed of earthly sins before it can return to the creator. They believe that a person's Karma is formed by his/her good and bad deeds. Karma controls what a person will be in the next life. In Hindu belief the human soul does not have to be reborn in a human body – it may be an animal. The wheel of life keeps turning until the soul is pure enough to return to the Spirit of Creation.

Good deeds alone are not enough to purify the soul in Hindu belief. Religious duties and rituals such as Yoga may also help. The Vedas are religious books of knowledge.

Unlike other world religions, Hindus are shy of organisation. The community therefore tends to take care of its own in a way that is not evident to those outside the community.

Worship

Most Hindus today are followers of one of the personal gods. The centres of worship are temples, but some worship takes place in the home. At certain times of the day the head of the family will make offerings and say prayers before the image of the god.

The River Ganges is regarded as sacred, with purifying and healing properties. Most Hindus wish to have their ashes scattered on the River Ganges after death.

Dress

Hindu women who dress in a traditional way will wear a sari over a short blouse and an underskirt. The midriff is usually left bare. The Bindi (coloured red spot on the forehead) may be worn by married women.

Most men wear western clothes.

Diet

This is very important to Hindus. They have a great love of animals because of their belief in reincarnation. Therefore, they do not believe in killing animals. A cow is the most sacred animal and the killing of a cow is a great religious crime. Hindus are very strict vegetarians. They will not accept food which has come into contact with prohibited foods. Practices differ, so ask the family of each Hindu which foods are regarded as prohibited.

Attitudes to illness and medical/care staff

Hindus will tend to favour the use of home remedies and will be slow to seek medical help. However, they will usually willingly accept the authority of the professional, either male or female.

Death and dying

Relatives may wish to bring money and clothes for the dying person to touch, for distribution to the needy. Passages from the Holy Book and prayers are said to the dying person. Threads of three strands (upanayana) may be tied around the wrist. The forehead is marked with holy paste. Relatives will want to wash the body and put on new clothes before it is removed. Traditionally the eldest son should take a leading part in this, however young.

It is believed that after death the soul immediately leaves the body to start its new life. It is the hope of every Hindu not to be reborn but to achieve unity with God. God's name is repeated into the ear of the dying person. Sometimes the dying person may request to be laid on the floor as they die.

Hindus are cremated as they believe that a body without a soul is a carcass. Cremation should take place before the next sunset. If the body is to be left in the room overnight a light or candle must be left burning throughout the night.

Islam (Muslims)

The followers of the religion of Islam are called Muslims. This world religion was founded by the Prophet Mohammed in Saudi Arabia in the sixth century AD. It is founded on two basic principles of faith:

• There is no other God but Allah. He is one being.
• Mohammed ("Peace be with him") is his prophet.

Muslims in the UK originate from various countries. The majority are permanently settled from India and Pakistan, or visitors from Africa and the Middle East. Muslims are found all over the world. The estimated population of Muslims in the UK is 1,500,000.

There are five pillars of religious duty:

• Creed (belief)
• Prayer
• Almsgiving
• Fasting.

Fasting takes place for the whole month of Ramadan, which falls at different times of the year because the calender is different from our western calender. During this month all Muslims must fast from dawn to sunset. The sick, the aged, children and nursing mothers are excused.

Pilgrimage

Once in a lifetime, if possible, every Muslim is expected to make a pilgrimage to Mecca, the Holy City of Islam.

Worship

The Mosque is the religious centre. Men and women are segregated into different rooms. All Muslims pray five times a day. The prayer itself is a set of rituals which are carried out while kneeling on a special mat and facing towards Mecca.

The holy Koran is the most sacred scripture of Islam. There is no priesthood: anyone who knows the Koran and the Islamic life can lead the prayer. This man is called the Imam (leader). Friday is the Holy Day of the week

Diet

Muslims are forbidden to eat pork or pork products. In addition a Muslim cannot consume the meat of animals or birds which is not ritually slaughtered (Halal). Towns with Muslim populations of any size will have Halal butchers. Alcohol is forbidden but not tobacco. Older people will tend to be more conservative about diet. It is advisable to consult the family of Muslim residents.

Dress

Free mixing of the sexes is forbidden in Islam. Women must cover their bodies, apart from their faces, at all times, especially in public. Women wear a head scarf and men a brimless hat.

Attitudes to illness and medical/care staff

A Muslim woman is not allowed to be attended by a male doctor unless a female is present, and generally it is better if she can be cared for by women.

Muslims believe that whatever happens, good or bad, can only take place with the consent of Allah. In adversity a Muslim is forbidden to despair and required to be patient, seeking help through prayer.

Death and dying

Muslims believe in the resurrection of the body after death, therefore they bury their dead rather than cremate them. Burial is expected to take place as quickly as possible. Before burial the body is washed and wrapped in a shroud. A funeral prayer follows when a relative dies.

Judaism

The roots of Judaism go back over five thousand years. There is no single founder of the religion but the prophet Moses is recognised as its most important leader. Jews believe that there is only one God and he is the creator. Judaism teaches that because God is good, so people should be good.

They believe that they were chosen by God as a people to be the "light to all nations". They do not try to make converts, and you have to have a Jewish mother in order to be classed as a Jew. The Tenachi is the oldest sacred book of the Jews. It is that part of the Bible which Christians call the Old Testament. The first five books are considered the most important; they are called the Torah. A Jewish religious leader is called a Rabbi. The estimated population of Jews in the UK is 300,000. Many arrived in this country in the 1930s as refugees.

Christianity

Christianity is the main religion of the UK and has more adherents than any other faith. It has different forms resulting from culture, nationality and belief. However there is considerable common ground between the different forms.

It is founded on the teachings of Jesus Christ who lived in Palestine 2000 years ago. Christians believe in the Trinity. This means that the one God has three aspects:

God the Father, God the Son (Jesus Christ) and God the Holy Spirit. Different traditions may emphasise one or other of these aspects.

The Holy Book of Christians is the Bible which includes the Old Testament (the same as the Torah of the Jews) and the New Testament (the teachings of Jesus). Christians worship in churches which have been built in almost every village and town in the country since the 3rd century AD. The more important places of worship are known as cathedrals. There are specially trained ministers or priests who lead the worship and care for the people.

The Christian church has seven sacraments, Baptism, the Eucharist (also called the Mass, Holy Communion or the Lord's Supper), Confirmation, Confession, Matrimony, Ordination of Priests and the sacrament of the Sick. Different traditions place emphasis on the importance of different sacraments.

The largest Christian group or tradition in the UK is the **Anglican Church** or **Church of England** (C of E). It includes the Episcopal Church of Scotland, the Church of Ireland and the Church in Wales. Fifty-seven per cent of the population of the UK are baptised as members.

About 13 per cent of the UK population belong to the **Roman Catholic Church**. Roman Catholics consider Mary, the Mother of Jesus, to have a more significant role than the other Christian groups do. They will only accept the ministry of a Catholic priest and might want to receive the Sacrament (Mass) as often as possible. (However you might find some Anglicans from the Anglo Catholic tradition whose worship would be similar to Roman Catholics). It is best to find out from the family which tradition they come from.

The **Free Churches** – Methodists, Baptists, members of the United Reformed Church, the Presbyterians and Moravians etc – are also a large group.

Many Black people of Caribbean descent as well as many people of white European descent are **Pentecostals**. Their worship may be led by a Pastor or a member of the congregation who knows the Bible well. They use free prayer, not following a set service in a book, and often focus on the gifts of the Holy Spirit. They may often talk about God speaking directly to them and express themselves in a manner which to outsiders, may seem to be strangely extravagant and colourful language. It must be understood that this is part of the culture, and should by no means be classified as a symptom of mental disorder.

Diet, dress and attitudes to illness and medical staff present no unusual features as Christians still make up the majority of the population and the culture of the UK has developed through Christianity.

Death and dying

Believing Christians of any denomination who are regular church goers will want to see members of their church community, or a minister or priest. The Sacrament for the Sick may be very significant to Catholics and some Anglicans. Some Roman Catholics may not agree with cremation.

You will be familiar with the customs surrounding death, although these differ in groups such as the Irish, Caribbean and Italian communities. When considering the Asian population we should not forget that there are many Christian Asian people in the UK as well as Muslims, Hindus, Sikhs and Buddhists.

People from minority ethnic groups are likely to want friends and relatives around them while they are dying. They will certainly want regular visits from their priest or minister. The residential home should make facilities available for this to happen.

Smaller Christian groups

There are many smaller groups such as the Quakers (or Society of Friends), the Plymouth Brethren, and independent Evangelical churches, which have their own culture about illness, dying and death.

Other churches or groups

It is very important to be sensitive to the beliefs of people who are Jehovah's Witnesses, Seventh Day Adventists, Mormons, Christian Scientists and others. They will mostly be cared for in residential care homes run by their own group but some people will inevitably end their days in secular places.

Again, the message is very simple. Find out as much as you can when the resident joins you, from them and from their family. If they seem likely to be terminally ill, find out what would be most helpful for them and for their family.

Points to remember

1. When someone comes from a different ethnic or religious group from us, it is harder but all the more important to find out all about their background – their culture, customs, tastes and preferences, and the things that are important to them.

2. The UK has always had immigrants who came to this country from other places throughout history.

3. We can classify people who come from minority ethnic groups by language and by religion.

4. When communicating with someone whose first language is not English, the use of interpreters is vital. It is not good practice to use other family members to interpret.

5. There is much more to communication than spoken language. We also need to interpret the culture.

CHAPTER 3

Communication

Karen Bryan, Jane Maxim and Tessa Perrin

> • *Talking and listening – with your eyes as well as your ears*
> • *Changes that come with the ageing process • Communication problems*
> • *How dementia affects communication • What to say – and how to say it*
> • *How to listen well • Non-verbal communication • Communicating*
> *with the person who is severely impaired*

Talking to people who have dementia is perhaps the most difficult aspect of care to get right. We can talk to them, but do they listen? And if they do listen, how much do they understand? This chapter looks at how elderly people communicate, and the differences between a number of specific conditions which can affect communication in elderly people. It then goes on to explore some special difficulties dementia brings, and how they affect two-way communication.

Communication is a process of conveying information between two or more people. It involves talking, listening, writing and reading. Before communicating there needs to be a thought, which is then put into words and sentences to convey meaning. The words are spoken using co-ordinated movements of the larynx, tongue and face to produce speech. But part of the message is usually conveyed by other means:

• hand and body movements to produce gestures, like shrugging the shoulders.

• changes in voice and pitch; for example we describe someone as "sounding" angry.

• the use of facial expression, such as a smile or frown.

The listener needs to attend to this information, as well as listening to the actual words spoken, to appreciate the full meaning. So listening involves using your eyes as well as your ears.

Being able to communicate with other people is a vital part of our lives. For many elderly people it is particularly important because limitation in mobility can restrict their daily activities.

For people with dementia, communication will be made more difficult by mental deterioration and resulting changes in behaviour. Before considering these changes however, it is useful to look at the effects on communication of normal ageing and specific conditions. These may add to the dementing person's problems with thought, memory and other mental operations.

Normal ageing

The process of ageing usually causes people to slow down, so that talking and understanding may be slower than in younger people. Older people also have occasional difficulty in finding the word they want. This is known as the "tip of the tongue" state; it happens to all of us sometimes. They also show differences in their style of talking. They may tend to give lots of details and perhaps even "ramble" a little.

But these changes in style of communication do not affect their everyday ability to communicate. It is therefore important that elderly people are given every encouragement to talk and to express their opinions. A lively, interesting environment will help to stimulate conversation.

Sensory problems

Many elderly people have difficulty in hearing and seeing. These problems can interfere with communication so it is vital that hearing aids and spectacles are prescribed, regularly worn and regularly cleaned. The person with a poor memory will need to be reminded every day about wearing and using these items.

Some people do not like wearing a hearing aid. An alternative which can be used for any resident consists of a microphone attached to a small amplifier. You speak into the microphone and hold the amplifier to the resident's ear. Most equipment catalogues for the disabled advertise these useful aids, and they are relatively inexpensive.

Teeth are very important for clear, understandable speech. Many older people have badly-fitting dentures or do not wear them, usually because ill-fitting dentures cause discomfort and even pain.

The importance of attending to eyes, ears and teeth cannot be stressed enough. Imagine yourself trying to have a conversation while wearing another person's glasses, with cotton wool in your ears and a large moving object in

Is the older person
• wearing cleaned glasses?
• wearing a hearing aid in good working order?
• wearing dentures that fit well?

your mouth. Try it and you may gain some insight into the problems that many older people have to cope with!

What else affects communication?

As well as the sensory problems of hearing loss and poor sight, certain specific problems can affect communication. These can include:
• dysphasia
• dysarthria
• depression
• confusion.

Dysphasia
This is a disturbance of the ability to produce or understand language; it may affect understanding, speech, reading and writing. The most common cause of dysphasia is a stroke affecting the left side of the brain. Many people with dysphasia also have some paralysis on the right side of their body but some do not, and these people, without any physical symptoms, are sometimes wrongly diagnosed as having some form of dementia.

People entering a care home may have had a previous stroke causing dysphasia. In general, the communication abilities of dysphasic people do not get worse, and some may show improvement if given suitable encouragement.

People with dysphasia have difficulty producing speech. For example, they might say "tea" meaning "I'd like a cup of tea" or "di" to mean dinner. Sometimes the person may make an error of sound, eg "do" for "no"; or a word error, eg "man" for "woman" or "he" for "she". Sometimes understanding can be well preserved despite the person's difficulty in speaking.

In other dysphasic people, speech is very fluent but not many specific words are used, so very little information is conveyed. For example: "Oh, yes, well you know, it's all very well, never mind." Someone with this type of "empty" speech may also have great difficulty in understanding what is said to them.

When trying to communicate with a dysphasic person, observe what the person can and cannot do. Try to note what is happening when the person does manage to communicate, so that you can provide effective help. The following guidelines are helpful to remember when speaking to a dysphasic person:

• Slow down your rate of speech.
• Remove distractions such as television which will interfere with listening.
• Break down your speech so that you give one part of a message at a time.
• Try to imagine what the person might want to say; using questions that only need a yes/no answer may be useful. For example: "Do you want to have a wash?"
• Give the person time to speak and answer.
• Maintain contact with the person while they struggle to find words; look towards them, look interested and wait patiently.
• Show sympathy if the person becomes upset or frustrated.
• Remember the person is not stupid; speaking very loudly and very slowly does not help. Use your normal voice and expression.
• Ask the person's opinion.
• Use gestures while you speak, and look out for their gestures and facial expression. For example, a person who mixes up "yes" and "no" will usually show which they mean by their facial expression.

• Dysphasic people are very aware of what is going on around them
• Try to talk to them as normally as possible
• Show sympathy if they become frustrated when talking

• Remember that speech is a great effort; do not expect a dysphasic person to talk for too long, and be alert to signs of fatigue.

Dysarthria

In dysarthria the nerve supply to the muscles used in speech is disrupted, so that production of speech is difficult. The muscles may be weak and floppy, making speech jerky with sudden changes in loudness or pitch. Muscles can also be unco-ordinated, causing speech to vary unexpectedly. This variation can cause the person to sound slurred or even drunk.

Dysarthria does not affect understanding of language or the ability to decide what you want to say. There is also no disruption to reading and writing skills unless there are other physical problems such as poor eyesight or weakness in the hand and arm muscles.

When communicating with a dysarthric person, it is important to allow them time to speak, to listen carefully and to watch for gesture and facial expression. It is often the case that people in everyday contact with a dysarthric person can "tune in" to their speech and understand them very well.

Some dysarthric people can produce very little speech, or their speech is unintelligible. It may be possible for the person to use writing, a communication chart or an electronic aid to help their speech or even replace it. You may need to contact a speech and language therapist to discuss their individual needs.

Depression

A significant number of elderly people have depression. Depression can profoundly affect communication, particularly the will to communicate. As well as showing little interest in events and their surroundings, the depressed person may not start conversations or respond when spoken to. Their speech will often be very quiet, with no variation in voice or expression.

All these aspects of depression may give the impression that the person is not able to communicate properly. Give the person time to communicate and accept whatever form of communication the person chooses. If you ask a question and they respond by nodding, then respond positively to that nod.

Confusion

A person may become confused because of acute problems such as a urinary tract infection, sudden admission to hospital or a drug side effect. This kind of confusion is temporary, and the person gets back to normal when the crisis is over, the infection treated or the drug stopped. But in dementia, the confusion persists.

Communication is affected by confusion in the following ways:
– reduced recognition, understanding of and response to the environment
– difficulty with recent and distant memory
– inability to think clearly
– confusion about where they are and who the people around them are.

Emotional impact

It is important to consider the impact on the elderly person of not being able to communicate normally:
• difficulty in expressing immediate wants, for example to go to the toilet
• difficulty in expressing feelings such as sadness, anger

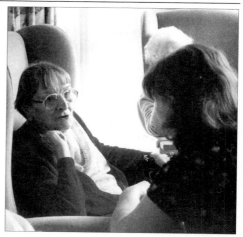

To communicate well, it helps to face the person and make eye contact on the same level. Use their name before you begin, and from time to time during the conversation. Touch may also be helpful, reminding them to listen.

• difficulty in expressing needs, for example to see a family member, or to write a will.

This leads to immense frustration, which is understandable, but it often gains the person the label of being "difficult".

Communication difficulty also affects relationships with other people – family, carers and friends, and can lead to social isolation.

Communication and the dementing process

As each person is a unique individual, quite different from anyone else, the way that person's dementia develops is also unique; no two people's difficulties or disabilities will be quite the same. However, there is a common pattern we can recognise, and focusing on a real person can help us understand how communication skills are progressively affected in dementia. On the next two pages you can read the story of the last few years of Ted Wallace (not his real name), who died recently at the age of 71.

Not all dementing conditions will be like Ted's of course, but if you have worked in dementia care for any length of time, you will be aware of much in Ted's story that is familiar. In it we can see many of the problems that can make communication difficult. You can see that they do not all come from memory loss, but include emotional, social and communication factors too:

• Ted found it difficult to keep tabs on what the time or the date was, or where he was or should be at any given moment. This led to cover-up remarks and defensiveness, in an attempt to hide his mistakes.

• He couldn't always remember things people said, or events that happened only a short while ago. Because of this he often repeated himself, or declared that these things had never happened in the first place.

• He didn't always understand what had been said to him, and would give a response that sounded all right to him, but which sounded very odd and out of place to the other person.

• He often couldn't find the right words to say what he wanted, and this made his conversation sound vague and woolly.

• He found that whereas he used to be able to think of and do three things at once, now he had trouble concentrating on even one.

• These changes frightened him; sometimes he would get very frustrated and angry trying to do things the way he used to; sometimes he would get depressed and give up, and withdraw into himself.

• His fears and his mood changes stopped him seeking out the company of his friends as he used to; sadly, it also sometimes meant that some of his friends lost interest in him too.

• As time went on, Ted gradually lost the ability to recognise the people and things that had once been important to him.

• He started to have real difficulties with language; he mostly lost the ability to converse, and relied instead on a small number of phrases or stories that for some reason stuck in his mind.

• Even these words and sentences later came to sound like gobbledegook, and eventually Ted stopped speaking altogether.

• Towards the end of his life, it seemed as if he had lost the ability to feel. His moods flattened out, and his face showed little expression. It was really hard to know if he was happy or sad.

The difficulties described here arise from a mixture of disordered speech, language, understanding, memory, mood and relationships. It is a very complex picture, but we must try to see it as a whole if we are going to communicate effectively with a person with dementia. The best approach will vary for each individual, but it is perhaps useful to start by considering how we communicate with someone both with words (verbal communication) and without (non-verbal communication).

Preparing to communicate

How can we best get a specific message across? Unless dementia is very far advanced, it is usually possible to do this if we prepare the resident in the right way:

• Face the person and make eye contact on the same level as the resident: sit if they are sitting, stand if they are standing.

• Use their name before you begin speaking, to make sure that they are attending.

• It may help to use their name from time to time in the conversation and to touch them on the arm or hand, to remind them to listen.

• Keep any background noise or distracting activities to a minimum (turn down the TV).

The person may have difficulty both in understanding what is said to them, and in talking themself. This means that any form of conversation is difficult for them. When we talk with another person, we usually look at them and use words which indicate that we are addressing that person. It is very important to make sure the resident is ready to listen or to talk. It is often quite noticeable that people with dementia do not look at the person talking to them. It is as if they have forgotten that this is one of the rules of conversation.

Another of the rules of conversation is that if you start off a particular topic, unless you indicate that the other person can change the topic, the other person will continue it. People with dementia often break this rule. They may know that they should respond to what you have said, but they have not understood what has been said to them. You com-

The story of Ted

Ted was 63 years of age when things started to go wrong. He had been the manager of a well-known DIY store for 24 years, the last 15 in the same local branch. His work colleagues were the first to notice changes. He had been quick-thinking and decisive, but now it was difficult to get him to make decisions, and he didn't seem to be able to hold on to the important parts of a discussion or argument. His secretary found he was missing appointments, documents were going astray, letters not answered. When challenged, Ted would say he had been overdoing it, feeling unwell, had just had flu... He started to take time off sick, and his doctor recommended a substantial break, maybe even a holiday abroad.

Ted did take a holiday, but it was a disaster. Though he and his wife Louise returned to their usual hotel in the Greek islands, Ted was restless and moody. He didn't seem to recognise familiar places and wondered why they had come. At his request they returned home early.

Ted was not able to return to work. In the end a diagnosis of early dementia was made and he took early retirement. Louise hung on to her part-time job for a while and tried to encourage Ted to take on some of the household tasks. He would willingly go shopping, but often came back with the wrong items, even things they never used, and Louise was never quite sure where all the money went.

After the episode of the flooded bathroom, Louise gave up her job. Now they were always in each other's company, their relationship became strained. Louise was irritable; Ted couldn't seem to remember what she had just told him, and would repeat the same question over and over. He could say what he wanted for dinner, or what he wanted to see on TV, but was no longer able to discuss the state of the world, or express an opinion on the news.

The gardening they continued to do together, and it gave Ted pleasure. It didn't matter if the occasional prize bloom was pulled up. He could no longer remember the names of plants, or how to use a trowel and hoe properly, but would often tell the same "Flower Show" story from their past. Louise would try to remember to laugh at the punch line on each occasion. In the end Ted would just sit and watch as Louise did the gardening; she preferred it that way, it was easier.

Some of Ted's friends were no longer in touch. Louise put it down to embarrassment. Bob and Vera still came though,

ment that the weather looks lovely today. Mrs B says that she wants to go home and where are her shoes? She has responded to your conversational opening but she has probably not understood what you said.

If you listen closely to what a person is saying, often the form of a sentence is quite normal and the words are in the right order, but it is specific words which are not right. In the early stages of dementia only a few words may be affected. Perhaps the person cannot remember names very well and uses pronouns (he, she, they) instead of the correct name. This can be very confusing; you may need to ask a question, for example "Did Jane come to see you?"

Sometimes the wrong word may be used but it may be close to the right word – "I want my eyes" instead of "I want my glasses".

Sometimes it is possible to build up a web of meaning to help the person. They may not understand one specific word, even if it is repeated, but if several words or ideas are used that have similar meanings or are all to do with the same topic, then understanding may be helped.

---

and were very supportive. Ted rarely recognised them now and usually greeted them, if at all, as new acquaintances. They never stayed long. Ted wasn't able to join in the conversation; sometimes he didn't seem to know they were there, sometimes he became agitated and abusive. But the visits helped Louise.

Louise no longer took Ted out with her. She didn't drive, and his agitation and shouting on the bus on the last two occasions had embarrassed and upset her badly. So she mostly stayed at home, where Ted now followed her every move, from room to room, even to the toilet. It seemed that if she wasn't directly in view, he would think he had been abandoned.

The only time off she got was when the homecare worker came and sat with him, and she would spend a few hours by herself. But the look of relief on Ted's face and occasional tears when she returned, made her feel guilty.

During the winter of Ted's 68th birthday, Louise's health broke. She spent three weeks in hospital, and a further month with Bob and Vera. Ted was taken into a residential home the day after Louise was admitted to hospital, and it was five weeks before she saw him again. Bob drove her over to visit him.

They found Ted in a chair in the corner of the room; he didn't recognise either of them. When she was able to return home, Louise started visiting every day. This seemed to make a difference; sometimes Ted would seem to recognise her and return her affection, but sometimes he wouldn't. He couldn't put sentences together any more, but conversed in a sort of gobbledegook that she couldn't understand, but she would try to join in. Occasionally he would give a one-word or one-phrase response appropriately to a question. "How are you today?" "Fed up!"; "How was the outing yesterday?" "Alright." But this happened less and less often.

Eventually Ted stopped speaking altogether, only making occasional noises. Louise would visit every lunchtime and feed him his dinner. It helped the staff a little, and it helped her to have something concrete to do. She could talk to him, hold his hand and stroke his hair, but most of the time his eyes were glazed and unseeing, and Louise felt that she might as well not be there. On rare occasions his eyes would meet hers and hold her gaze, and then Louise felt that he knew her, that there was a thread of communication between them, and was glad she had come. Ted died just before his 71st birthday.

What to say

Here is an example of a carer talking to a resident first thing in the morning and trying to help that person get orientated to the time of day:

Mrs Jones, good morning.
Did you have a good night's sleep?
It's time to get up now.
You can get dressed and then you
can have your breakfast.

Here is another example of a carer talking to a resident about her son:

Mrs Jones, your son Tim has just rung.
Tim is coming to see you tomorrow.
It is Friday today and tomorrow, on
Saturday, your son Tim is coming here.

Note that the carer has used the son's name, Tim, rather than "he".

Sometimes presenting a limited choice is helpful. First introduce the topic and then give the person the choice:

Would you like a drink, Mrs Jones?
Would you like tea or coffee?

How to listen

Misunderstandings can happen between residents and care staff quite easily. Try to work out what the basic message might be, and don't take what has been said as exactly what the person wanted to say. Above all, don't react with abuse if you are verbally abused, however hard it may be to stop yourself. The resident will usually calm down much more quickly if you speak calmly and gently.

As an example of listening to the underlying message we will consider the resident who says that something of theirs has been stolen. They may mean that it is missing, or that it has been moved, or even that they are confused about what is happening.

In early stages of dementia, when the person may be aware that their ability to function and think is changing, they

Coping with verbal abuse:
• Speak calmly and gently
• Think about what the person may really be trying to say
• Don't contradict

may be depressed about these changes. If that person is already a resident in a home, they will need particular care and reassurance at this time.

The way you say it

In the later stages of dementia the person may not understand the specific words that are being used, but you can convey a general message. This message is conveyed not by what you say but how you say it. The resident may well be able to pick up the emotional content of the message through the rhythm of your speech. You can put across sympathy, anger or firmness just by the tone of your voice.

This point may also be very important if you have any residents for whom English is not the first language, and if there are no staff who can speak the person's language. Facial expression and tone of voice can convey a great deal.

Helpful responses

It can be difficult to know how to respond sometimes, and what to say, when a person with dementia says something odd or inappropriate to you. One useful way is to try to see through the actual words they say to the feeling behind them. For example, if someone says "I must go home. I've got to get dinner for the boys," you could reply, "You sound anxious about your family, Doris. Are you missing them?" Chapter 4 will guide you with helpful approaches.

But even with your very best efforts,

there are likely to be times when your response to something a resident says will make them puzzled, frustrated, or even angry and panicky. After all, if you truly believed your family were at home waiting for you if only you could find the bus stop or undo this latch, wouldn't you be devastated if a stranger told you that you had to sleep here for the night, in a building you don't recognise, with people you've never seen before?

Sometimes we are lucky, and say or do something that seems to help and calm the person. The better we know the person, of course, the more likely we are to get it right. But for those difficult times, when we are finding it hard to stay calm ourselves and just don't know what to say, a few pointers might help:

• Prevention is better than cure. Get to know as much about the person as you possibly can.

• Try and ensure that the person has a busy, enjoyable day. If you can make your unit somewhere it's a pleasure to be, conflict is less likely in the first place.

• If a reality-orientating approach seems to upset the client, don't use it.

• Humour is a great de-fuser of emotional tension.

• Distract from the immediate conflict with something you know they like: a cup of tea, a walk to the shop, a hairdressing session.

• Try to make sure that your home or unit has places and signs they can recognise, so that it not too difficult for a person to discover where they are, or how to find their way about.

While on the subject of anger and hostility, we need to recognise that *you* might be the one developing these feelings. To be asked the same question repeatedly by a client for hours on end can tax even the most patient person. To be accused of things you haven't done

or said; to be the butt of another's grief or anger; to be sworn at, abused or perhaps even hit – all these things are the occasional lot of the person who works in dementia care. Knowing that it isn't directed at you personally doesn't always help. Sometimes it just hurts; sometimes you want to retaliate.

Part of being a good care worker is knowing your limits, knowing when to walk away, knowing when to ask for help. Never be ashamed to acknowledge that you have reached this point. A good manager will be sympathetic and give you some breathing space.

Non-verbal communication

For the dementia carer, non-verbal approaches are probably the most powerful communication tools we have. They are important at all levels of dementia, and become increasingly so as the condition advances.

Touch
Touch is critical; it is after all the most primitive form of human contact. For the visually impaired person, or the person with severe dementia who is unable to make eye contact, it may be the only route we have. Find out, if you can, how the person liked to be touched in the past. Was theirs a family used to lots of hugs and cuddles, or was it reserved, giving only pecks on the cheek in greeting? This will give you a guideline.

If you have no means of obtaining such information you will have to work by trial and error. Try a stroke or a squeeze of the hand, a touch of the hair, an arm round the shoulder. Most people find this kind of contact acceptable, and if the person doesn't like it, they will find a way of letting you know – they will pull away, or express displeasure on their face. In this way you will gradually learn

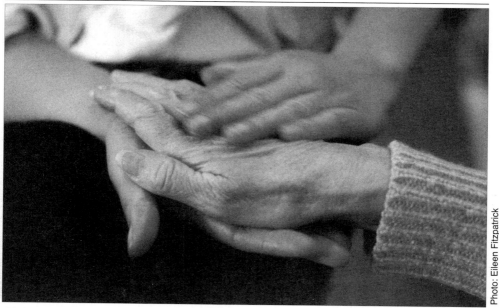

Photo: Eileen Fitzpatrick

Sitting with someone with advanced dementia, giving them your full attention, is probably one of the hardest, yet one of the best things you can do. Giving a hand massage as you sit, can help.

what the client needs – a full-blown hug, to walk hand in hand, or perhaps to have their back stroked.

A colleague of mine once planted a spontaneous kiss of affection in the middle of her client Arthur's forehead. He sighed deeply and she suddenly worried that she had done something unacceptable. "My mother used to kiss me like that," he said. A small but very important piece of knowledge that she could then build in to her individualised care.

Body closeness

Don't be afraid to come close. The more impaired the person is, the closer you will need to be to establish communication. Don't stand and speak from six feet away and expect the very impaired person to respond. It may feel like invading their personal space, but barriers and territories are disrupted in dementia; the rules have changed. It's likely that you will need to come close, probably to come into physical contact.

Body orientation

Earlier in dementia, where some insights and abilities are still intact, sitting side by side or at a 90-degree angle to each other is generally comfortable and companionable. Face to face can feel threatening, so avoid it if you can. However, in later dementia the rules are disappearing; eye contact is very important, and face to face may be the only way of obtaining it. With the severely impaired person, position yourself at their level and in the line of their gaze.

Remember too, that in your approach to a person, it is always a good policy to approach slowly and from the front. Never rush in quickly and never from behind or from the side. With people who are blind or who have impaired sight, you must take even greater care.

Posture

Try to be relaxed; if you are tense other people can sense it easily. Lean towards the person.

Gesture

Don't be afraid to use gesture as you speak; then you give the person a double chance of getting hold of your meaning.

Facial expression

It is difficult to know how others see us; we are not usually aware of the expression on our face. But make a conscious effort to smile (particularly if it doesn't come naturally). As you talk with someone, try to reflect in your own face the emotions you are picking up from them.

Eye contact

Try to make eye contact at the start of any communication; it is very important. Try to understand which emotions the person is conveying, through the expression in their eyes.

Voice

Think about the qualities of your own voice, and listen to other peoples' voices. Which voices are easy on the ear; which do you want to hear more of; which do you want to turn away from? Make a conscious effort to use your voice in a sensitive way. Try to reflect in your own voice, the tones you are picking up from your resident.

Communicating with a person who is severely impaired

Of all groups within our society, there can be few more socially and emotionally isolated than those who are far advanced in their dementia. Recent research has shown that most severely impaired people in institutional care spend little more than eight per cent (around about an hour) of their waking day in any kind of social interaction; for some it is a lot less than this.

Staff and time shortages play their part of course, but the biggest problem seems to be the discomfort many care staff feel when faced with someone who cannot communicate in words. Carrying out a task such as feeding or bathing a client doesn't usually present a problem; the difficulty arises in communicating without a task to fall back on. "What can I say? What should I do? Won't I look silly if I talk to them and they don't respond to me? Won't I look even sillier if they respond with a stream of gobbledegook and gesture which I don't understand, and don't know what to do with? Does it matter anyway?"

Yes, it does. People who are unable to start off social interaction are the most in need of our time and our help. If you have felt this kind of discomfort, take heart in the knowledge that you are far from alone. We have all felt like this at times. But it should not stop us from trying. One of the most important tasks we have as carers, is learning how simply to "be" with our clients; not doing this or that necessarily, not seeking any particular response; simply letting them know that we are there for them, that we are available, that this is time to be shared. Our full time and attention is probably one of the hardest, yet one of the most valuable things we have to give.

The next time you have 15 minutes to spare, go and sit with one of your more impaired clients:

• Sit at their level, make eye contact if you can, and some form of physical contact if it seems appropriate.

• Talk to them, and if you run out of things to say, it doesn't matter. Learn how to be comfortable with a companionable silence.

• If your resident responds to you with noises, or perhaps with their own kind of special language, listen carefully.

• Listen as much for the emotional tones as for understandable words and phrases. Be aware of gestures and facial expressions that accompany the communication.

• Listen actively – nods, smiles, mmms and uh-huhs – your own non-verbal signals. It tells the person that you are in touch, in harmony. Don't let your gaze wander, don't look at your watch.

• Listen reflectively: try to mirror the emotion that is coming through. If the communication seems to be about something humorous, laugh and smile; if it looks as though it is supposed to be shocking, be surprised; if confiding, act as though you are sharing a secret; if angry or grief-stricken, crumple your own features into a similar pattern.

• Respond in words if you want to: "You're frowning May. You seem to be very cross. And you're shaking your fist. I shake my fist when I'm angry. I wonder if you're angry too?"

Reflect, mirror, respond. It says to the other person that you know where they are coming from, and that you appreciate how they are feeling. It is possible to have a long and very satisfying conversation without a word of conventional language being spoken. Give it a try.

Try not to run away

If your resident cannot respond vocally, don't let that chase you away. It is very hard to stay with a situation in which you feel you are being quite ignored; but try to stay with it. It is quite likely that you are the only means these residents have of warm human contact. All the principles so far discussed still stand. Try to stay in physical contact and in eye contact. Talk to the person as far as you can.

Try a little hand or neck massage while you sit with them; it might help you to feel you are doing something useful. Is there a cat about who enjoys an undisturbed lap; or a cuddly dog? Is there a

favourite song? Would the family know of any familiar music? Can you bring a small cassette recorder nearby? If you have the confidence, sing to the resident. Sometimes we just need to be less self-conscious; we are likely to be of more use to our residents if we can.

Uncharted territory

You may discover responses as you put some of this into practice; you may not. Each individual is quite unique; no two people, no two dementias, and to be honest, no two ways of communication are quite the same. Much of the time, we do not know what we are dealing with.

This is uncharted territory; very little research has been carried out; very few therapies have been applied. Answers are only going to come as we work through our fears and feelings of inadequacy about working with people who have dementia. With patience and commitment we can achieve communication, make relationships, and take risks with our own emotional vulnerability.

The challenge before us is this: we must learn to speak and understand the language of dementia.

Checklist for good practice

1. Communication is vitally important to the wellbeing of the person with dementia, and it depends largely on you.
2. Listening to them, giving time, care and attention, lets the person know you are in touch.
3. If you show by your facial expression and patience that you are thinking about what they are saying, or communicating to you, they will know you are trying to understand them as an individual.
4. Just being there with them lets the person know you care.

CHAPTER 4

Taking communication a step further

Bob Woods

• Good interaction between staff and residents tranforms the quality of care
• Discovering the individual and their life story • Truly individual care plans
• Reminiscence therapy • Discovering meaning: listening with care, time and
attention • Responding in a helpful way • Validation therapy and resolution
therapy • Discovering potential and developing skills

In the previous chapter, the foundations of good communication were discussed. Care workers need to develop skill in using these important building blocks – verbal and non verbal – in day-to-day practice. The impact can be far-reaching.

Good interaction between staff and residents transforms the quality of care provided. Personal care that is carried out in silence feels insensitive and even rude to the person, whereas if you talk to them about what you are doing, you can convey warmth and gentleness. Good interaction helps in building up relationships, helping staff to see each resident as an individual, with a unique pattern of responses and preferences. Staff who become skilled at interacting (especially those who develop their listening skills) become more aware of the individual needs of those with whom they work.

Developing relationships

In this chapter, the emphasis will be on extending communication beyond the first social contact, and beyond the purely task-related interaction, towards levels of communication where relationships develop and flourish.

This appears to be the most difficult aspect of communication for staff to enter into readily. Often it seems there simply is not the time to spend with residents "just talking". Sometimes this is a throwback to the days when talking with residents was not seen as "real work", when staff were made to feel guilty for not busying themselves with such essential tasks as cleaning out cupboards or sorting the laundry.

There are always more jobs to be done, of course, and never enough staff. The issue here is whether or not spending time with residents is seen as an important part of your work, as it should be.

If all else fails, there is the time you spend with the person during physical care. The interaction here does not have to be confined to the task – a relaxed bath-time may be an excellent opportunity to get to know the resident. Many homes have a key-worker system, but unless the key-worker has allocated time to spend with the resident, they cannot begin to fulfil this vital role. The reality is that many staff find developing interaction a very demanding task. Unlike physical care tasks it often feels that it can be put off till later, and so it tends to be avoided.

The effects of this neglect may not be instantly clear, but the damage is done nonetheless. Without close human contact residents remain withdrawn, with their feelings locked in, or have to try to make contact in ways which become labelled as "attention seeking" or behaviour problems. Staff become immersed in physical care, and lose out on the satisfaction of being part of meaningful dementia care. However, those staff who commit themselves to developing their communication skills soon find there is much to discover.

Discovering the individual and their life story

Every resident will have a unique life-history, which will have contributed significantly to their current situation, their manner, their interests, their concerns, as well as health, cognitive impairment, personality and social support. (See also chapters 1 and 5)

Some life events are shared with many others of the same generation, but each individual's experience of the same event will be different. For example, many current older people lived through the Second World War, but each will have had their lives shaped, enhanced or scarred by their experiences quite differently. The world has undergone huge changes in the person's lifetime, which are hard enough to keep pace with before the onset of any cognitive impairment. How much do we know or understand about the person's life story, about

the events and relationships, the achievements and disappointments that have mattered to that individual?

Awareness of the person's life history, a biographical approach, is important in communication for several reasons. Firstly, it will help staff make sense of the resident's perhaps incomplete attempts to communicate; helping staff fill in the gaps enough to keep the channel of communication open. Often family are able to make sense of something the person is trying to say which has mystified the staff, because of their greater awareness of relationships and events in the person's life. The better you know the person, the easier it is to understand him or her.

Playing to their strengths

Secondly, many people with dementia can get to their store of long-term memories much more easily than their memories of more recent times. By talking with someone about past experiences, you will be playing to their strengths, drawing on long-term memories, some of which will be well-rehearsed, some of which will have been embellished here and there over the years, some perhaps not brought to mind for many years.

You will be able to communicate interest in and respect for the person, placing the person in the position of "expert", as their knowledge is (for once) superior. The person has lived through times that you have only read about or seen on archive film. As your awareness grows, you will be able to prompt the person more effectively to talk about different aspects of their lives, and access more of the range of long-term memories stored over the years.

This process will be greatly helped if "prompts", such as copies of family photographs, significant objects or items of clothing from their past, are available. Sometimes it is possible to work with the

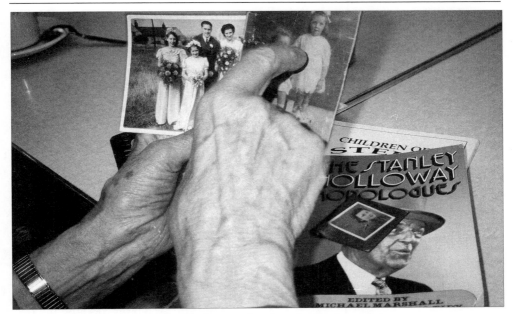

Reminiscence will be greatly helped by "prompts" such as family photographs.

person and their family to produce a life story book for the person. This would typically consist of an album, illustrated with photographs, depicting the main events and relationships of the person's life: birth-place, early family, schooling, first and subsequent jobs, marriage, family, places lived, holidays, retirement, grand-children and so on. A book like this is a powerful aid to communication, helping the resident to share readily with new staff something of their life.

Truly individual care plans

Thirdly, care plans (see chapter 5) will be vastly improved if they are based on an understanding of the person's lifetime of interests, preferences, priorities and ways of coping. In this way care plans do actually become individualised, and responsive to the individual's needs. A care plan is devised for Mrs Jones, rather than for a dementing person at a certain stage or level – for a real, whole person.

The care plan will reflect important aspects of the person's life story – their interest in music, the close relationship with their grand-children, their long service in the church choir or whatever – adapting the activities and roles according to the person's current ability level. Thus Mrs Jones' care plan might include participation in a weekly hymn singing session in the home; having a special noticeboard devoted to photographs and news of her grandchildren in her room; staff ensuring that she has access to her favourite music, perhaps on cassette on a portable machine, or sitting with her in her room while she listens.

Reminiscence therapy

Here I have described a particularly individual, biographical approach to what is often called reminiscence therapy. Reminiscence is also often used in group work, with the aim of opening up communication between the person with dementia and other residents, as well as with staff. A wide variety of memory triggers are commercially available – objects and pictures of everyday life, stars of stage and screen, royalty, news events, music and archive recordings, video-tapes and so on. These are a good starting point, but it is well worth making the extra effort to obtain more local material, and material especially relevant to the resident(s) with whom you are working. As well as families, local libraries and museums will be valuable sources of help in identifying and obtaining copies of useful reminiscence discussion starters.

A few words of caution are needed regarding reminiscence approaches:

• Be careful of making assumptions about the person's experiences, based on how we imagine we would react in similar circumstances. Let the person tell their own story, and avoid putting words into their mouth. This can be difficult with residents who talk little; it means we must be tentative in our prompting: "That sounds a very upsetting situation. How did you feel when..?"
• Some knowledge of relevant history (both of the local area and the wider world) can be helpful to place memories in context, flesh out some of the details and so on, but not to *correct* the person. You are not giving a history lesson, but trying to encourage sharing of personal memories.
• Be sensitive to the person's reactions. People will vary in how much they wish to share of their lives, and how much they wish to keep private. It is important to respect the person's boundaries and not to appear to them as over-inquisitive or intrusive.

For many, there will be areas of pain and hurt in the past, not fully resolved. Beware of allowing these areas to be exposed in a group where it may be difficult to give the individual immediate support; and when working on a one-to-one basis, check out with the person whether they do wish to talk about the matter further with you.

Discovering meaning

Taking communication further involves listening more extensively to what the resident with dementia is saying. In the past, there was a tendency to dismiss the person's efforts at communication as rambling and confused. However, it is now recognised that behind the words which apparently do not make sense, there may be an underlying meaning, which represents an important effort at communication. This means that care workers need to listen even more carefully, in order to try to discern the hidden meaning, and certainly not "switch off" because the person seems confused.

Communication is of course concerned with conveying and receiving information. However, there are a variety of types of information involved. For example, as well as information that is task related and factual, there is information that tells a story, information that reflects the person's feelings and emotions, and information that serves a social purpose. A conversation between two close friends might not involve the exchange of much factual information, but convey feelings of warmth and express the social need that each has for human contact.

Many interactions convey meaning at a variety of levels, and usually – but by no means always – people find words which together with their non-verbal communication express their meaning to their satisfaction, judged according to the particular situation and listener. The person with dementia may be in a situation where the underlying motive for the communication still arises – the feeling, the need, the discomfort – but the "appropriate" words do not follow. Instead, other words and phrases come out, or the emotion triggers recall of fragments of an experience or story, which sound like nonsense to the unaware listener.

Discerning the hidden meaning can be difficult; at times it will be far from obvious. It's important to tap into all the sources of help that are available:

• Invite the person to elaborate by showing your interest in what they have to say, communicating your attention non-verbally through eye-contact, facial expression and head movements, making encouraging noises and comments such as "go on", "tell me more".
• Don't interrupt the person's flow. Listen patiently if they are slow, avoiding the temptation to cut in, finish the person's sentence or to correct statements that (from your perspective) are "wrong".
• Listen with your eyes to the person's non-verbal communication, which may tell you more clearly than words about the person's feelings.
• Hold in mind the person's life history, which may help you piece together what is being communicated.
• Try to look at what is happening from the perspective of the person with dementia. Try to stand in their shoes, with an open mind, preferably leaving your own personal hang-ups behind! How does the world look from their angle?
• Be sensitive and careful in reflecting on what the person has said and in probing further. For example you might say: "It sounds like you're talking about a very unhappy time for you"; "Was anyone else lost with you?"

Clearly this level of listening requires concentration, and the listener has to clear their mind of other concerns, being fully available for the person. If they only have half your attention, the moment will be lost.

Your response

How you respond to the hidden meaning will vary greatly according to the situation. But the important principle is to respond to the person's underlying feeling, rather than getting too involved and hung up over the words used.

The following interactions show how this principle works in action:
R = Resident, S = Staff member

R: (calling out to care worker) Help, help, let me out, I've got to get home!
S: You're very upset, Mrs Jones. Who is it you're worried about?
R: It's Jean, she doesn't know where I am, and she'll be back from school.
S: Tell me about Jean - she's your daughter isn't she?
R: Yes, and if I don't get to her soon, there'll be hell to pay.
S: Being with your family is really important to you, isn't it Mrs Jones. I think I saw some photographs of you all together in your room – shall we go and look for them?

R: Who are all these people? Who invited them in? Look, they're drinking my tea? They shouldn't be here, this is my home...
S: Who would you like to have round for tea?
R: Just my parents and people from church, but I don't know these people, get them out of here...
S: You sound really angry that these people are here sharing your things; shall we go to your room and make sure your private things are alright?
R: Yes, they'd better be under lock and key with these people here...

In the first example, the hidden meaning seemed to relate to parental concern for a daughter's well-being; in the second, the resident is perhaps expressing her need for privacy and to have her own possessions, and the difficulty of living together with a group of "strangers".

There can be no prescribed, universally effective responses, of course; every person with dementia, every interaction has unique features. But what these examples have in common is that they do not deny or invalidate the strong feelings the resident has; the resident's feelings are real feelings. The staff member does not say "Don't be silly – your daughter is grown up now" nor seek to reassure the person before acknowledging the depth of feeling being experienced. The staff member is accepting and respectful, not dismissive, judging or devaluing.

Listen for the feelings

Approaches which seek to listen and respond to the emotional content of the person with dementia's communication have been described as **validation therapy** or **resolution therapy**. The main difference between these approaches is how much the emotions expressed now are thought to reflect unresolved conflicts from the past.

In the first example, a validation worker might suspect that there had been a time when Mrs Jones' daughter was small that Mrs Jones had felt she had let her down by not being there when she was needed; so that now she must be with her at all costs. In the second, perhaps the resident had been attacked and robbed in her own home, and so now felt especially suspicious of strangers and their motives. In each case a worker using resolution therapy would be as likely to suspect a recent event as one from the person's distant past.

There is no real difference in technique involved here, simply one of emphasis. The wise worker will perhaps reflect that people with dementia find themselves in extraordinarily difficult circumstances, and that there are many current sources of stress and conflict to add to those which most of us accumulate in our journey through life.

Discovering potential

One of the rewarding aspects of extending communication with people with dementia is that we begin to see that the person has abilities and capacities that no one thought were there. Staff have a key role in helping residents to have the opportunity to participate and communicate to their full potential.

Imagine a team game of some sort, where some players are really skilled and others are beginners. The shape of the game depends entirely on the attitude of the skilled players. They can show off all their skills, and let the beginners get by as best they can; or they can bring the learners into the game, feed them straightforward passes, and guide them through the trickier parts, using their additional skills to make sure everyone can stay in the game. It is likely that before long in the first scenario, the beginners would withdraw from the game; in the second, they are much more likely to gain pleasure and enjoyment, and even develop some skills of their own.

In dementia care, staff are fortunate in having numerous skills and abilities which dementia has denied to many residents. Running verbal rings around residents is easy, but, of course, pointless. It is much more satisfying to keep the residents "in the game", not letting the conversation go over their heads, but bringing them into it, making it simple for them to respond, supporting them when they are finding the going tough.

Helping communication

How can we make it easier for residents to communicate? The following list may be a useful starting point:

• Create a social atmosphere. We all feel readier to relax and talk in a comfortable, homely place, rather than in an area like a large clinical "waiting-room". Refreshments appropriate to the occasion act as social lubrication!

• A small group size encourages more participation and more sharing of experiences. Group work with people with dementia can be very rewarding, and a number of more detailed accounts of the issues involved are available (see further reading list).

• A shared task, activity or outing encourages communication. Part of the reason for the low levels of interaction in some residential homes is that there is simply nothing to talk about, because nothing ever happens!

• Small children and pet animals (both carefully supervised) visiting the home will often stimulate much interaction.

• Appropriate music adds to the social atmosphere, encourages reminiscence and interaction.

• Memory prompts – photographs, personal mementoes, a newspaper, magazine, information boards and such – help the person converse without putting so much strain on memory. Focusing on something you can see and touch makes communication much clearer.

• Supporting the person in taking on meaningful roles helps the person experience a sense of purpose. For example, in validation groups, one member takes on the role of music leader, another welcomes the other group members, another serves the refreshments. As the person takes on the role they also take on a reason to communicate, rather than simply conversing for the sake of conversing.

• Stimulation which captures the attention of the person with dementia, perhaps through multi-sensory input, may also form a talking point. For some highly aroused residents, calming stimulation – relaxing sounds/music, peaceful light effects, for example – helps them to be calm enough to be able to concentrate and communicate more clearly.

Different residents will of course respond to different situations. Many people with dementia communicate much less than they are capable of, because the circumstances they are in do not encourage interaction.

New learning
Many people with dementia are in fact capable of some learning and development; some, especially those with milder impairment, learn to use memory aids and prompts. They need to be able to trust the information they are given, and not to hear different messages from different staff; otherwise they will learn that it is useless to seek answers (or will seek them more and more desperately).

Confrontation, telling the person repeatedly they are wrong, is clearly not a helpful strategy; it may well fix the person more firmly in their mistaken idea. Responding honestly but sensitively to the person's questions, helping them to find out relevant information for themselves, is an appropriate use of **reality orientation**, which has become associated with an emphasis on correction, but at its best was an attempt to help the person with dementia to achieve their potential level of function.

Both reality orientation and validation emphasise the importance of honesty in the responses of staff to residents; sometimes it appears that a "white lie" would save everyone concerned a great deal of upset. It is a good golden rule for staff not to lie or deliberately mislead residents; greater confusion can result, and the person's adulthood is devalued.

The truth, but not always the whole truth

However, clearly in any interaction we do not necessarily tell the "whole truth" (life is too short). We tell only that which is necessary, relevant and appropriate at the time. Thus, if someone is talking about their mother, it may not be essential to talk about the mother's death, if the hidden meaning relates to feelings of security, and a response on this feeling level appears appropriate. There is then emotional truth, without necessarily needing to go into the truth of chronological, factual history.

It is conceivable that there may be exceptions to the golden rule of honesty, but this would need to be agreed and implemented on a team basis, taking all the individual circumstances into account, and seeking external advice before following a pathway of deliberate deception.

A wider view

Finally, it is worth noting that much of the content of this chapter is not really specific to dementia. Most of us communicate better in small groups, respond to a social atmosphere, enjoy some nostalgia, and do not always make the emotional content of our communication crystal clear. What we all need to do is use our vast experience of human interaction and communication and apply it to the special needs of people with the disability of a dementia.

Checklist for good practice

1. Spending time and talking with residents is an important part of the care worker's job. Time *can* be found to talk, and talking changes a physical task into a person-to-person contact.
2. Awareness of the person's unique life story helps staff to understand and communicate more effectively, and to develop more responsive individual care plans.
3. Communication involves listening not just to the words spoken, but also to the feelings and meanings that lie beneath the surface. The person's body language and life history give clues to hidden meanings; active listening is required.
4. Responding to the hidden meaning opens up new avenues of communication.
5. People with dementia often function below their potential, because they do not receive the sensitive, flexible support they need. Getting to know the person better as an individual will assist greatly in adjusting their environment and our approach so that they are able to function as well as they are able.
6. Confrontation is seldom a helpful approach. Deliberately deceiving residents cannot be recommended as an alternative. It is possible to be selective and sensitive so that honesty in the interaction can be retained.

Further reading

Holden UP, Woods RT (1995) *Positive approaches to dementia care* (3rd edition). Churchill Livingstone, Edinburgh.

Feil N (1993) *The Validation breakthrough: simple techniques for communicating with people with "Alzheimer's-type dementia".* Health Professions Press, Baltimore.

Gibson F (1995) *Reminiscence and recall.* Age Concern England, London.

Stokes G, Goudie F (1990) *Working with dementia.* Winslow Press, Bicester.

CHAPTER 5

A living plan
for care

Joan Costello

*• Try to walk alongside the person with dementia, to see and understand the world
as they are experiencing it • Welcoming a new resident into your home
• The importance of observation and listening skills • Care planning that is
person-centred • Rights and risk taking • The care environment*

If we are committed to attaining the
highest quality of life for each person
in our care, this commitment will
shine through their Living Care Plan.
When we think about how someone is
introduced into residential care we need
to place ourselves alongside that person,
to look at that person's life and walk with
them on the road which they might have
planned for themselves.

The trauma of change

For almost all people who live in this
modern world, the most significant feature is the rate of change of everything
that surrounds us. Technology, our physical environment, our social lives and perhaps our moral outlooks, are features
that would not have been recognised
even a few decades ago. Changes for
some can be for the better, but for others
the world has moved on too quickly, leaving them uncertain and confused. This
then is the picture for you and me as we
get older.

People with dementia (and those who

display symptoms similar to dementia)
find change particularly difficult to cope
with. Many of them appear to live for
most or all of their time in yesterday's
world, or more probably in a muddled
series of yesterdays. They may be grasping
at the happenings of half remembered
days of long ago.

The world which surrounds them now,
the places, the people, the events, may
not match the pictures in their minds.
They may not recognise the place they
are in, or know how or why they are
there. They may be unable to use the
knowledge of what they are seeing or
hearing, to determine where they should
be going, or what they should be doing.
For many, damage to their brains has
been aggravated by the stress of living in
our society or by the nature of their circumstances. In addition there is the slow
deterioration which comes with age.

Other people may have no physical
damage to their brain, but have been sub-
jected to stresses of life which they were
unable to cope with, and now show characteristics similar to those of dementia.

Once again their condition may be complicated by the processes of ageing. As in dementia, the person's choice of action may appear to be quite illogical.

Whatever the cause of the condition, all people with dementia have one thing in common. They all need our understanding. For the care worker, the importance of the clinical diagnosis of the person's condition is insignificant compared to knowing how to provide help and care.

Moving to a new environment

A change in circumstances or environment can be difficult for many of us, even though we can fully comprehend where we are and what circumstances brought us there. A person with dementia may be unable to understand where he or she is is going or why, or even if they understand at the time, can't hold on to that knowledge.

For many it can be a frightening time. Strange people and unfamiliar surroundings may provoke a feeling of insecurity. A clean white tablecloth can be quite forbidding to someone used to eating from a wooden kitchen table. The need to go to the toilet can be quite disastrous to someone who is unable to make his or her desires known.

"Why am I here? Who are you? I need to go home," are familiar words from a new resident, and sometimes from someone who has been with you for a long time. Remember too that it is unlikely that the person with dementia made the decision to go into residential care themself.

Amid all this turmoil they may be desparately trying to anchor their fleeting sense of themself, and clinging to the last remnants of what is familiar to them. People who they may not even recognise are telling them "what is best for you". The change to the new environment can become a frightening experience for many and one from which it may be difficult to recover.

The key to easing the pain and fear is good preparation, which must contain certain vital components. So the person or persons who are to do the assessment must be well prepared.

There must be genuine respect and understanding of the person's damaged world. It is so important to search for and see the real person underneath, not the one which may appear on the surface. How would you feel if you were living with dementia? Try to put yourself in their shoes, and see the world as they are experiencing it.

Think carefully about the complex and intense feelings they must have, involving their partner and other family members.

On a practical level, we also need to find out how the person manages with their dementia in their own home. Their ability to cope, even though this may be limited, is something that we must preserve. This must eventually be prominent in the care plannning.

Planning for the move

Although your responsibility for care really begins at the time of admission to the residential home, there is much to be done before that date. Planning begins, or should begin, before the first contact is made with the person living with dementia.

Let's see how that works, in a residential or nursing home setting.

It is assumed that before the first visit, the head of home will have received medical and social reports and will have invited the close relatives or carer to the home for discussion. Staff will have told them then about the philosophy and facilities of the home, what it can and can't do, and the carers or relatives will have talked from their point of view about the person with dementia. It is again assumed that the head of home will discuss with you all aspects of this meeting. Outline planning will very much concern itself with the preparation of the care worker who is to accompany the head of home or senior for the visit.

Every contact with the person – staff visiting them at home; them visiting the care home; contact with family, friends or neighbours – will yield useful information. All this information should be added to build up a profile of the person with dementia, and fed in to the preparation of their care plan.

Prepare yourself

Remember that most, if not all, of your experience of dementia will have taken place in the atmosphere of a residential home. It can be quite different meeting for the first time someone you know very little about, in an environment far removed from the home in which you work. It is vital that you, as keyworker, are well prepared for the assessment/admission process so that you appear relaxed and confident, and can give all your attention to the person. Interruptions and distractions should be discouraged, and you must try hard not to get caught up with other tasks in hand, but have total commitment to the resident.

Discuss all aspects with your senior. Be certain that you are both on the same wavelength.

Be prepared to listen. This visit is not the time for you to air your own views.

Confidentiality must be observed at all times. Whatever you may see or hear, or be told, it is never to be discussed with anyone other than staff who are directly involved.

Think about what you will wear, and about how your appearance, and what

you say and do, might be viewed by the person with dementia and their relative or carer. Try to look unthreatening: no uniform, no pens and notepads.

The welcome should be relaxed and informal in order to prevent a feeling of intimidation or that the staff are "in charge". The person may be intimidated or give quite the wrong impression of themselves to somone who seems to them to be in authority.

Making the first visit

While it is important not to delay the first visit, it is equally important that the timing is acceptable to the family member or carer. Meet the family and the potential resident without preconceived ideas. You may have read previous reports, the opinions and views of other professionals. At this stage disregard them. Don't be tempted by labels or the well-turned phrase which others may have produced. You need to try hard to meet the person and the carer with an honest openness and interest, freeing yourself and them from any inhibited views which may create barriers to communication and forming a relationship.

We have discussed only the situation of the person coming from home into care, but of course they may be in hospital or another residential home. Wherever the visits are made, your skills of observation and constructive listening are most important.

Observational skills

The observation of one person by another needs to be a two way process. It is just as important for the person living with dementia to see and get to know you, as it is for you to observe them. Every observation needs a purpose. On this occasion our purpose is to determine whether this is the right time for this person to enter residential or nursing care. Remember though, that it is the affected person who should be making that decision and not the family member(s), and so an important part of your observation is to try to determine their true feelings.

All observational exercises must include the following guidelines (but this should not be taken as an exhaustive list):

Does the person:
• Appear to be happy or disturbed?
• Make efforts to be friendly?
• Seem to be in control of themself?
• Appear to live in the present or in parts of their past life?
• Has he or she retained personal abilities? Observe dress, hygiene and organisation of the living environment.
Does he or she:
• Relate and interact with other family members, with their partner, neighbours or any others present?
• Show fears or anxieties?
• Have carers or family members who are able to continue with care? Do they seem to be under stress, showing signs of distress or deterioration in health?
• Does the person recognise the stress caused to others?

Take stock of the home environment and of those things the person looks upon as essentials. Study the layout of the room. Which items and their positions in the room, appear to be particularly significant. This information will be vital when preparing for admission. Many things which you see may not appear to be of value, but they may be of exceptional importance to that person. Little bits of jewellery, a watch, perfume, a handbag or purse, even moth balls may be things that the person clings on to and may feel lost without.

Above all, are there any things which are, or have been, sacred or special to the person during his or her lifetime? A bible perhaps or a prayer book, a cross or rosary, a musical instrument or maybe just an old letter.

Pets should be accepted provided that they can be accommodated. Cats and dogs in a home can create a homely welcome and opportunities for extra love and care. Visiting PAT dogs (see *Resources*) should be encouraged; for residents who like them they can bring the sensory pleasures of stroking, hugging and reassuring a live animal. Caged birds or a well-kept aquarium also provide company and stimulation.

Listening skills

However powerful the onslaught on your other senses, what you hear is of paramount importance. The stench of the place may be overpowering or the visual scene horrific, but you must not let this distract you from listening. The picture you are going to remember and write up is made up of what you have seen, what you have smelled and what you have heard. Of these, the last is the most important. Hear and read (through the non-verbal messages too) the feelings and anxieties the person is experiencing.

If your listening is to be constructive, you must attend to what the person says, not the comments *you* have made. When you come to write up your account of the conversation, the important part is what the person said; not what you said.

• Switch off your own inner thoughts.

• Have total interest in whatever conversation takes place.

• You will need to ask questions and you may only have a limited time.

• You may have to guide the conversation, but remember that this must not lead the person away from his or her own thoughts.

Sometimes the person will not be easily understood. There may be unfinished sentences ending in garbled sounds. Respond always as if it were a normal conversation. Maintain eye contact. Try to pick up what the person is feeling and trying to say. Read the body language (see Chapter 3). The person may repeat statements or questions. Listen and reply as if it is the first time you have heard them. For the person with dementia, it is the first time.

It is very important not to give the person the impression that they are incompetent, nor must they be allowed to feel excluded from the conversation. Any discussion between yourself and family members must include them, not be conducted over their head. Remember too that the person with dementia is an adult and not a naughty child, even though some people may talk in those terms.

Avoid discussion out of earshot of the person. This can promote paranoid thoughts of being talked about, and may cause anger, mistrust and low esteem. Above all, your listening must never appear to be judgemental. Listen carefully to everyone present, and allow them to feel they have been heard, but remember that the most important voice is that of the person with dementia.

Vital admission procedures

Where possible both the person with dementia and their carer should be invited to the home before admission. This needs to be done on a friendly basis, to share a meal together and meet other people. The invitation to a meal is something which the person can focus on. It is not wise to have the person sitting in reception, in an office or having a conducted tour of the home.

Good communication is vital. This means that the person with dementia, the family, the staff team and other professionals must be kept informed. All information must be documented and made available to all team members, keeping always within strict confidentiality.

Prepare the person's room with the help of the family or carer. Try to imitate the environment of their room at home. Pictures and photographs should be hung or placed where they always were in relation to a bed or chair, not where you think they look best.

Position the bed so that it is familiar. Think of which side the person is used to getting in. Did it face the window? How many pillows? Blankets or a duvet? Has the person been used to a commode or even a bucket? Above all the person must be helped to recognise and acknowledge that this is their room. But this does **not** mean repeating the words, "This is your room". It is better to use the information which you have, or should have gained, to provide clues both visual and verbal to enable the person to accept the new surroundings.

New residents must be asked whether they would like their own name on the door of their new room. It must not be assumed that this is the person's wish just because it is the standard practice in your home. Very few people have their name on the door in their own house. However, the number or name of a house they remember with fondness (not necessarily the one from which they have just come) may provide some feeling of home, so it may helpful to put this number on their door.

Does the person have any special dietary needs? Have the kitchen staff been advised? Have supplies been obtained? Are there any special nursing, chiropody or dental needs which the home will not be able to provide? Has the district nurse been told? Has the person been registered with a local GP?

Time of arrival

Key staff must be present. This must include those members who did the home visits.

Try to maintain a calm and welcoming atmosphere. Make sure you have time and space to be with the person and minimise any distress and confusion. It could be traumatic for resident and family if the key worker has to be called away.

Be sure that everything you may need is available. Does the person need a wheelchair, for instance?

On arrival

After they have become familiar with their new surroundings, allow the new resident to make his or her way around the home, but accompanied by a carer if necessary. Do not leave the person alone in bewilderment.

Avoid overloading the person with questions like, "Where did you live before you came here", from each new member of staff on duty. A better approach is to make conversation familiar by using details already known. For example, "It was lovely meeting you at your house/the hospital…" "How is your daughter?" "I liked your garden" This will give the person a sense of being recognised and remembered.

Anticipate the questions or requests that the new resident may make. "I must go home now" "Why am I here?" "No one knows me here."

Acknowledge the loss and bewilderment that the person is feeling. Put aside any thoughts of "They are always like this to begin with, but they usually settle down in a few days". Now is the time the new resident needs the understanding which you have been trained to provide. Give them the time and opportunity to express themself. Listen to their requests sympathetically and act on them wherever possible. Replies will be different for different people, but examples could be: "Moving and settling in to a new place is never easy" "We are very glad to have you to stay here with us" "This is a home where many retired people come to live" "Many of the people who live here have difficulty in remembering" "Your doctor feels that it would be good for you to stay here".

Avoid statements which are deceptive or untrue. They give nothing to the person with dementia; their only purpose is to get you out of a spot. All responses must be honest, but honesty must be delivered always without causing hurt or pain to the inner feelings of the person. It is vital for us all to develop our skills in recognising just how much truth of their situation and condition the person can cope with, at the particular time of their question.

Personal profiles

Putting together a profile of the person begins with the first meeting and is added to, as our relationships with the person and the family develop.

The profile is intended to inform us about the person's life. It must provide information on people, places and personal attachments that the person will talk about. This will include information on childhood, education, occupation, hobbies and any other details of the person's unique personality.

The profile should aim to present the picture which the person would wish to present for him or herself. Profiles are best structured from information first gleaned from the person then linked together by family or friends. If for instance the person talks of Bill repeatedly, find out from family or friends, who Bill is. Remember that we all should have the right to keep to ourselves those things which are personal to us and which we would not want the world to know about. These rights should not be denied to the person with dementia. Particularly where information comes to light and is shared with staff by the person with dementia, this must be respected and guarded.

Put people into care planning

Everyone's initial care plan must include:
• Ways of helping the person to settle into long-term care, in partnership with family and friends
• Planned time to listen to the needs of the resident
• An agreed approach towards understanding the person.
• Additional statements and amendments based on observation of the person's ways of coping with the changed mode of life.
• Physical needs must be recorded, specifying ways of preserving individual choice and dignity. For example, wherever possible it is much better for just one care worker to be involved in personal care, because this encourages a feeling of partnership between resident and care worker. The presence of two staff members will detract from this and put staff in control.

Bring the plan to life

Care plans should be regularly updated, read and used by the whole team. A care plan which is not used like this is a dead piece of paper – and the kind of neatly written care plan that lists date, problem, aim, resources etc has, in my view, very severe limitations.

Bringing a care plan to life means relating it to the person's life. It must therefore feature the following:
• A focus on people, residents and families, rather than problems
• A focus on abilities, personality, need of

love, sens
swear, etc.
coping fra
• A focus o
self determi
you agree o
person's poi
their immedi
• A focus on
past life of th
childhood, th
life's joys and ..hat do they enjoy, and what do they dislike? Who do they remember and how did these people influence their lives. Living care plans will sensitively recognise and reconstruct the human journey and promote an inner peace.

If you are successful with your care planning, this inner peace will be shared by the person living with dementia, the family, and you, the care worker.

Taking risks

Risk has two basic elements. The first is the probability of an event occurring. The second is the consequence of that event. Set in the balance against these two features is the right of every person to exercise their own freedom of choice of action. Precautions taken to make a disaster less likely, or its happening less destructive, may well erode the freedoms which we have a right to expect. A locked front door will take away our rights of freedom of movement but may lessen the probability of an accident on the road (see chapter11). Absolute freedom from risk is impossible. Even to approach total safety would mean a complete restriction of any freedom of action.

We must therefore look carefullly at each predictable situation and consider:
• What is the probability of an accident or other undesirable event occurring?

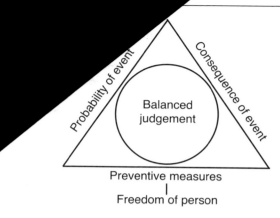

Probability of event / Consequence of event

Balanced judgement

Preventive measures
|
Freedom of person

In each predictably risky situation staff must weigh all the factors of risk and freedom in the balance and make a judgement – but that judgement will never be infallible.

- What will be the likely outcome if such an accident or event does occur?
- What precautions can we take and what effect will these have on the freedom of particular people or on the home in general?

In making our judgement we need to consider how the reasoning of people with dementia is different from our own. A person with dementia may not appreciate that the kettle is hot simply because steam comes from the spout.

Remember always that in weighing up all the factors of risk and freedom in the balance you are making a judgement, sometimes a best guess. No judgement is infallible. You will not always be able to predict events, but skills obtained from experience and observation will be a great help, as will discussion with other members of staff and other professionals. Above all what ever action you take about risks, this must be recorded and regularly reviewed. When caring for people with dementia, things can change from day to day and from hour to hour.

In the care home environment you will have the advantages of:

- Facilities with fewer risks to safety than the average domestic dwelling.
- Routines and disciplines designed to avoid accidents.
- Yourself and your colleagues who are trained to care and make decisions most appropriate to whatever situation is likely to occur.

Against these advantages, you will have a number of people with dementia living together. This may provide your greatest source of risk. Wherever people are obliged to live together, some will always fall out with others. Residential care for people living with dementia is no different, but control of feelings may be less inhibited.

You must develop the courage to allow your residents the maximum freedom of action. You need to balance the risk taken against the quality of life you are trying to promote.

Access to rights

Rights for everyone are always there, either in law or in the expectations of all of us to benefit from the things around us. What we do not have is a total access to our rights. Those of us who are blessed with a reasonable amount of intellect and may be quite vocal have obvious advantages over the less articulate in obtaining our rights.

People with dementia have the least access to their rights. In almost all cases their access has to be gained through some other person – a care worker, a family member or advocate. People with dementia can almost invariably express their desires in some way, but are unable to take the next step to secure their rights. Within the residential setting a great deal of responsibility for preserving a person's access to their rights falls on the staff. A simple desire to go for a walk, to the shop, to the hairdresser or to the pub, may not be acceptable to family members or convenient to the staff. The spending of a resident's money can often be viewed differently by different parties, family members and staff for example.

It is most important that the person is helped to retain, wherever possible, the access to rights which they held before the onset of dementia. A living care plan will always reflect these rights. Above all, the care worker needs to make the person with dementia feel that they still have all of their rights intact. The greatest impact on a person's feeling of well-being is the impression that no one listens or understands. Remember too that the person has the right to say "No".

There is a tendency among some people to think that because residents with dementia have an impaired intellect and less ability to communicate their needs, their needs are unimportant. This is perhaps understandable, but it is quite wrong. The desires and needs of people with dementia are still there, and if we look we may recognise their importance.

A person with dementia may not have retained the skills of hiding the external signs of emotion. They are no longer actors as we often are, putting on a show to please our audience and getting our reward. They are truly honest. What they show is what they really feel, which may not be the display we expect them to present. We must learn to recognise their needs. Above all we must never consider them to be of lesser importance or lacking the intensity of our own feeilings. They have equal rights with us, to have their feelings recognised and their needs fulfilled.

Rights in a community setting

For all of us, the exercising of our own rights nearly always diminishes the access of others to their rights, although gener-ally we also exercise courtesy and consideration so that others are not inconvenienced. Always though, our right to be at the front of the queue, when we can, means that others must be denied that right.

From our position of power as care staff, we must look at all rights through the eyes of the person with dementia. We must strive to help everyone in our care maintain access to their rights and achieve their desires. We also have a responsibility to exercise for that person the courtesy and consideration for others which they would have shown, but may not now be able to achieve.

The care environment

Our environment is our surroundings – place, people, objects and circumstances . In considering the environment in the context of dementia care the following definition may be more helpful: "The sum of external influences which affect a living body".

For as long as can be traced, mankind has had an instinctive desire to shape his environment. The rolling of a stone across the mouth of a cave, or the building of some form of dwelling, continues into the development of communities and cultures.

Security and safety were obvious reasons for this development, but alongside this was the need to define the space, either collectively in family units, or as individuals. With this came a desire to personalise the space, with distinctive buildings and decoration. This is strong, instinctive behaviour: wherever a person lives shows the stamp of that individual. Rows of identical new houses rapidly take on a personal identity. Prison cells, uniform from the outside, very soon relect the personality of the prisoner inside. Even hospital beds with their neatly fold-

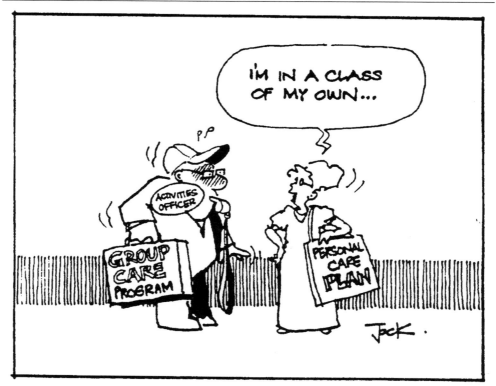

Cartoon from Rethinking Dementia, Ausmed Publications, Victoria, Australia.

Living care plans, regularly updated, read and used by the whole care team, will focus on the individual's sensitivities, beliefs and past life, what they enjoy and what they dislike.

ed blankets become places of identity and personal space. Books, flowers, the dressing gown, advertise who lives there. The immediate area surrounding the bed is often thought of as "My space".

The value of personal space is paramount in a long-term care setting, but it may often be overlooked. The centre of the home to the resident may not be the lounge or the dining room, or even their own room. To many housewives the focal point of home would have been the kitchen. This is where they may have sat with a cup of tea and a biscuit when they wished to relax. Does your kitchen have a few chairs and a table?

It may seem contradictory, but personal space is often a place to be shared. Some people living with dementia, who have lost so much, often find the need to be close to someone. They may have no vision of the future and have nothing left but the comfort of their fellows.

A settee in a residential home will allow two residents the comfort of close personal contact with each other, or for a resident to feel the security of a member of staff or relative sitting with them. Single chairs may not allow this. Simply to provide personal space, one's own room, and an easy chair, is not enough. Space alone does not replace the fulfilment of a life shared. Many, many people with dementia have died in their own space, in the utter loneliness of isolation.

Because someone is "contained" in pleasant surroundings it is easy to think that their needs have been met. It is important that those with dementia are enabled to exercise their own choice of things which will define their environment as they wish it to be. To surround them with the things that we ourselves think they need or what we think they should have, is not likely to promote a sense of well-being. The decor may be pretty and tasteful but the space still be a vacuum if feelings, impressions and acceptance are missing. The picture in the mind which the person with dementia constructs from the images surrounding him or her, may be quite different from our own impressions, and may be in conflict with remembered places of comfort and security.

Environment-centred care is no substitute for person-centred care.

Orientation

"Where am I?" "Where do I go?" These are familiar words to staff. Many people with dementia will spend hours trying to find some familiar reference point. A door to get out or a door to get in. Each new day may be a new experience of where they are. Because this is where they were yesterday does not mean that it is the place remembered, or where they think they are, or where they wish to be. It is very often the case that when a person with dementia moves to go somewhere, the objective (the place that they wish to go to) does not fit with the landmarks which surround them at the time.

The actual time of day may not coincide with what the resident thinks they should be doing. It does not help to persist in telling a person with dementia that it's tea time, if he or she is convinced it is some other time of day.

The person living with dementia will have brought their own environment in their mind from where they came from, and often from the distant past days of their life. Look for the clues that the resident will use, and build on these. Watch to see what the person recognises and may find significant in deciding which way to go or what to do next. Go with the flow of the person and not with the flow of residential care.

Toilet doors may be better left open, if that helps someone to use the loo when they need to. Better to have an open door to aid recognition than take another step towards incontinence and even destroying the person's self sufficiency.

The position of the bed, particularly in relation to the window, may be crucially important to the resident.

Try to provide clues which will help to show the time of day. A table laid for breakfast with marmalade, toast and cornflakes is more likely to provide the feeling of morning than an announcement that it's eight o'clock. The morning newspaper may tell the person what day it is. Drawn curtains, softer lighting and a warm milky drink mean evening and bedtime to most people.

I have found that it is seldom beneficial to have the resident's name on the door, or a photograph of the person. Many will read the name or recognise the picture, but won't make the necessary connection that this is their room.

Making the choices they have always made

Good orientation will enable people to make the choices which they have always been used to making. Orientation is not just about finding one's way about, but must include enabling the person to select the things he or she prefers. When offering a meal, show the person what items of food there are and ask whether they like whatever it is. Do not ask from the region of the trolley, "Would you like carrots", and hope this has been understood. Show them to the resident, saying "Would you like carrots?"

Record your observations, and include them in the care plan. For example, the lady who has always had her hair done on Tuesday, or the chap who played darts on a Friday night, should be enabled to continue with this routine in order to orientate them within their week.

It is vital that all team members are able to move out of their own safe and comfortable position and get into the surroundings which the resident is relating to, and from which they draw their own feelings of safety and comfort.

There are no simple answers to the problems of orientation. Landmarks are often exclusive to one person only and may not be readily apparent to the care staff. Probably none of the residents living with dementia in a residential home will be orientated to the present day. Even if they are, they may be desperately trying to return to an earlier age, reliving the feelings of their former role and the control they held over their life. Staff must be able to walk the resident's road, following their signposts in the period which they have selected. The most important thing in care is to recognise each resident's way of coping and to enable them to continue in the way they find comfort.

Discover what the resident is doing, or trying to do, and go forwards from there.

Above all, look, listen and learn.

Checklist for good practice

1. A change in environment or circumstances, like moving house, is stressful for all of us, but much more so for the person with dementia. Try to understand their fear and insecurity; above all listen to them, and respond with warmth and reassurance.

2. Building up a personal profile, and a living care plan that is regularly updated, read and used by the whole team, is most important.

3. The person with dementia has rights (for their needs and desires to be met) like anyone else, but they depend on care staff to secure them. In other words, their freedom of choice and well-being depends on you.

4. Most residents with dementia are not orientated to the present day but to an earlier time when they had a clear role and control over their life; from this they draw feelings of safety and comfort. The most important thing in care is to understand each individual's internal reality, recognise how it helps them to cope with their present predicament, and enable them to continue..

Resource

PAT Dogs (Pet Aided Therapy Scheme), Rocky Bank, 4 New Road, Ditton, Kent ME20 6AD. Tel 01732 848499.

CHAPTER 6

Mental health in older age

Dr Daphne Wallace

• What is normal ageing? • Physical, psychological and social changes • Illness in old age • The importance of recognising and treating depression • Schizophrenia of late life, neurosis, alcohol and drug abuse • Delirium or acute confusion • Alzheimer's disease and other dementias

Normal ageing is not an illness in itself but a slow biological process which affects people differently and at different rates. Illness is more common in old age and can make the situation much worse, but with active treatment much of this can be overcome. Modern units specialising in the treatment of elderly people have, one hopes, laid to rest that dreaded phrase, "It's just your age". Ill health and disability may be more common in old age, but they are not necessary parts of growing older.

Physical changes

"Normal" changes with increasing age are well recognised. The need for spectacles and false teeth is more common; joints become a bit stiff with wear and tear; hearing and balance are less acute. Loss of mobility or hearing may lead to social isolation and severe deafness may cause such feelings of isolation that the person is driven to feelings of suspicion and even open hostility.

Old age in itself does not normally lead to death; death is usually due to a failure of a major system in the body due to illness. Ageing leads to a reduction of the body's natural capacity to cope with problems, whether from outside, such as infection or injury, or from the inside such as blocking of one of the arteries supplying the heart.

Normal ageing leads to some loss of nerve cells in the brain. Confusion that comes as a result of physical illness is more common. Certain forms of dementia also are more common in old age. Other organs are also less adaptable. Thus the liver and kidneys may be less efficient at getting rid of waste products from the body. Elderly people are less able to adapt to extremes of temperature. We still do not know why some people age much more quickly than others. Some of it is due to our genes. It is often said that if we want to ensure a long life we should choose the right parents!

Psychological changes

The psychological effects of ageing have been much discussed. Most people show a gradual reduction in the ability to learn new facts or take in new situations from the mid-twenties onwards!

Ageing does not bring about psychological loss – only changes, some of which are beneficial. Older people may have more difficulty in abstract thought and may find they are slower at moving from one task to another. They need time to absorb what is happening and do not like to be rushed. Do not give them several different instructions at a time!

Social changes

The most significant social change in this century has been the increase in the percentage of elderly people in the population. Alongside this has been a reduction in the numbers of middle aged people who are able to look after them, as a result of both smaller families and greater mobility throughout the world.

Loss, in various forms, is a common experience. Besides loss of nearest and dearest there are other losses in day to day life. In the past the older generation were seen as the storehouse of accumulated knowledge and experience; a wise authority to be consulted for advice. Now modern technology brings the book and more recently the computer and the micro-chip for storing information.

In this, as in so many other ways, the older generation may find themselves without a role in society. Loss of status is important, but other losses are significant too: loss of income, health, independence, security of accommodation, all are stresses which many find hard to cope with.

Personality

An individual's personality does not change in healthy old age. The interaction of that personality with circumstances and events, however, makes the actual behaviour and attitude of the individual unique. Like anyone else, elderly people do not like to be treated as a group. Person-centred care thus becomes vital, as other chapters in this book have explained. For example, some old people like to join groups, some do not.

Illness in old age

Illness in old age can be physical or mental, but as we get older there is an increasing tendency to suffer a mixture of the two. Minor physical illness in older age often causes a sort of delirium when the person becomes confused or disturbed until the underlying illness is treated. Someone who is already confused may become more confused, even when suffering from influenza.

Physical illness

Acute illnesses which are most common in old age are heart disease, such as heart failure or "coronary" heart attacks; chest infections such as bronchitis and urinary infections. All illnesses are more common with increasing age.

Chronic illnesses are quite common and often more difficult to deal with. Chronic chest diseases or severe arthritis can be very disabling and lead to much distress.

Physical illness of any sort is especially difficult to assess in those suffering from dementia. They may be unable to tell people about their symptoms. Listening to the chest or doing routine urine tests therefore take on more significance. The fact that a person is old and may have dementia is not a reason to sit back and do nothing. Treatment may relieve suffering even if it does not bring a cure.

Mental illness

Mental illness or psychiatric illness occurring in elderly people may be divided into the following groups:
• those with functional psychiatric illness (no known physical cause) such as:

depression (the most common)
drug dependence
alcoholism
neuroses such as anxiety, and
all other types of psychiatric illness
found in younger people.
• those with delirium or toxic confusional states - causing acute symptoms of brain disorder
• those with chronic dementia from various causes.

Depression

Depression is the most common of the functional illnesses. Depression is a mood that we all know from time to time. Severe depression is an illness, requiring medical forms of treatment, counselling or psychotherapy.

If an old person, whether or not they have dementia, seems distressed or anxious, or slow, unhappy and unable to enjoy things, they may have a depressive illness. Different things may make this more likely: biological (in their genes), psychological (due to some stress or difficulty) or social (loss or change in their circumstances, such as admission to a home). In older people the important thing is to determine what are the main causes for that individual. Talking to them, and more importantly listening to them, is your role.

Severe depression affects at least three per cent of old people. If one includes milder depression, which still needs help, this rises to nearer fifteen per cent, so quite a lot of old people have this illness. One of the commonest first symptoms is loss of interest, and inability to enjoy things. Loss of appetite and subsequent weight loss may also be an early symptom.

Thoughts may be affected as well as mood and the person may begin to worry about money, illness, real or imagined, or ideas of guilt. In severe depression thoughts of worthlessness or fears about illness may lead to suicide. Many who are depressed develop anxiety symptoms and there is a danger that the agitation or anxiety may be treated instead of the depression. Depressed people may have marked slowing up and inability to perform everyday tasks. Dementia may be suspected but "pseudodementia" (the name given to this situation) should always be thought of so that the depression does not go untreated.

The presence of dementia does not prevent a person becoming depressed. Early dementia may make the person depressed, and it is always very important to recognise the presence of depression so that treatment can be given. Psychotherapy is more difficult when the person cannot remember things, but counselling can be used to good effect (though it may need much repetition).

Antidepressant drugs are very effective for the majority of people. Newer antidepressants which are safer in old people have made it easier to treat them safely. In a very few cases the symptoms are so severe that the wait for the drugs to work is too dangerous. Electroconvulsive therapy (ECT) may occasionally be used.

Other functional illnesses

Mania, the opposite of depression, also occurs in elderly people. It is less common than depression, but some people have an illness called **manic depression** where their mood may go "up" or "down". This needs specialist treatment

Very severe mood disorder can lead to symptoms including delusions (false beliefs); these are called **psychotic symptoms.** The person may believe they are so wicked that they are going to be arrested or that they smell or are rotting inside, for example. These symptoms can also be treated. They do not mean the person is "mad" and to be shunned or laughed at.

Schizophrenia of late life is much less common than depression. The person may develop ideas that they are being persecuted, commonly accompanied by hallucinations. (Hallucinations are false sensory perceptions. They may be sounds or voices [auditory hallucinations] or visions – such as the "pink elephants" described in alcoholic poisoning.) Treatment with medicine is frequently very effective though the sufferer may need to remain on it for the rest of their life. Unlike schizophrenia affecting younger people, it may not interfere with the old person's ability to relate to others and live in the community successfully.

However, if an old person is suspicious it does not necessarily mean they have schizophrenia. Our society sometimes treats old people in a way likely to make them have little trust in those around them, especially those in authority.

Neurosis used to be thought to be uncommon in old age. It is true that some neuroses of earlier life do resolve with ageing, but many neuroses just become more effectively hidden. Some neuroses start in old age. This may be as a response to stresses to do with ageing.

Neurosis is an unsatisfactory way of coping with the stresses of life. Thus someone may feel "safe" if everything is clean, and have to wash repeatedly. In elderly people the most common neuroses are of the anxiety-depression type. These occur in one third of all physically ill old people.

Marked **hypochondriacal** symptoms – being convinced that there is something wrong with the body all the time – usually indicate an underlying physical illness or severe depression. Bereavement may lead to a variety of problems including more severe depression. Dependent people may adapt badly following bereavement, and develop depression.

Alcohol and drug abuse do occur in elderly people. In women, problem drinking becomes more common with ageing, though it declines in men. An older lady who asks several times a day for "a little sherry" may have been taking too much for some time. About half of alcoholics in old age have had a lifelong problem but the remainder, mainly women, develop problems in response to stress.

Drug problems in older people are different from those in young people. They usually involve prescribed drugs such as tranquilizers or sleeping pills. Side effects such as confusion and falls are common. They may be taking a handful of pills at a time! Withdrawal effects may also occur if they are suddenly stopped.

Delirium

Delirium, or acute confusion, is due to a failure of system(s) outside the brain, producing temporary changes to brain function and consequent confusion. Acute confusion in an old person should be investigated immediately. Many treatable conditions may cause confusion. The most important ones are infection and drug side effects. Early diagnosis and treatment can prevent long term damage. Other causes include heart failure and dehydration. In the presence of dementia a very trivial physical problem such as a cold or constipation may cause a temporary sudden increase in confusion.

Dementia

What is dementia? It is not "just senility", it is an illness. Unfortunately it is common, affecting about one in five of the population over 80. (That means that four out of five people *do not* suffer from dementia) Dementia is a gradual failure of the functions of the brain. This can happen at different rates and in different areas of the brain at different times. Various conditions cause this deterioration. Some of these are: Alzheimer's disease, vascular or multi-infarct dementia (hardening of the arteries of the brain, in common language), dementia in Parkinson's disease which is now thought to be linked with Lewy body disease, and other causes.

Alzheimer's disease is a physical disease which causes a gradual loss of the ability to remember, to learn, to think and to reason. It is the commonest cause of dementia. About a half of all cases are due to Alzheimer's disease. The cause is not fully understood. A genetic cause has been discovered in a small number of families and there may be a genetic "factor" in other cases, but there are probably several different factors involved in most cases.

The illness involves certain changes in the brain which can be seen under the microscope. These are commonly known as plaques and tangles. Tangles are due to protein abnormalities in the brain cells and plaques are due to deposits in the brain of another abnormal protein called B-amyloid. The brain cells die.

The onset is usually very gradual and at first difficult to distinguish from forgetfulness due to depression, stress or normal ageing. The loss of short term memory is an early and striking sign. As the illness progresses, disorientation in place and time – sometimes leading to day-night reversal – and wandering become more common. Later, the thinking process becomes more affected and simple, practical tasks, like putting on clothes, become impossible. The person may not know how to walk or sit. The course of the disease varies. In some it takes many years to develop whereas in others progression is rapid. At present there is no known cause, though work is going on to develop drug treatments. Some drugs have now been licensed in the UK for the treatment of mild to moderate Alzheimer's disease, but they do not stop the disease process.

Vascular dementia, sometimes called multi-infarct dementia, is so called because *infarction*, or death of brain cells, results from interruption of their blood supply, either through bursting (haemorrhage) or blockage by a clot. High blood pressure can cause damage to walls of vessels which may then burst. Multi-infarct dementia occurs by itself in at least 10 per cent of cases and also occurs in combination with Alzheimer's disease. About 20 per cent of people who have strokes develop changes in mental function. Repeated small infarcts or strokes cause dementia.

The onset is often quite sudden, but may be gradual. Progression is often by a series of "steps" where there is a rapid deterioration followed by some improvement but eventually a further deterioration follows. People with this type of dementia often retain an understanding of what is happening to them, even when the dementia is very advanced. Physical signs of a stroke may or may not be seen, especially early in the disease. Treatment is limited to measures to control blood pressure and drugs (anticoagulants or aspirin) to stop the clots forming.

Dementia in **Parkinson's disease** and **Lewy body disease** is due to a different type of change in the brain cells. An abnormal protein (ubiquitin) accumulates in the cells and forms the Lewy body – named after the man who first described the changes. When Lewy bodies accumulate in the deep part of the brain which controls movement, Parkinson's disease, with its typical tremor, stiffness and stooping posture, develops. The side effects of some drugs can cause a similar picture.

A small proportion of people with

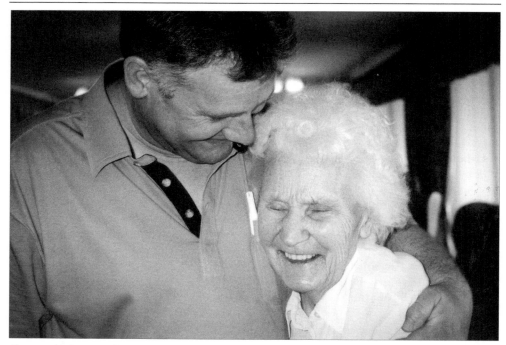

Dementia is an illness which gradually destroys the person's ability to remember and communicate; but it does not destroy the person inside.

Parkinson's disease develop dementia. Some may have changes of Alzheimer's disease but more commonly Lewy bodies are found in many areas of the brain. Common symptoms are visual hallucinations, variable confusion, frequent falls or other signs of muscular problems. This Lewy body dementia may develop with no obvious sign of Parkinson's disease.

Other causes of dementia include Prion dementias such as **Creutzfeldt-Jacob disease** (CJD). This group is very rare. They are now thought to be due to a particular kind of infective particle. These diseases do not appear until long after infection occurs – a long latent period. They are not easily passed on. They are usually rapid in progression once the dementia starts. New variant CJD (linked with BSE in cattle) occurs in younger people and progresses over months rather than weeks.

Dementia of frontal type involves the frontal lobe of the brain which is involved in control of emotions, judgement and behaviour. Injury or other damage to this area of the brain causes marked personality change without the memory changes seen in other dementias. This can be especially difficult as the person may feel quite normal but have changed ways of dealing with situations and people.

Huntingdon's disease is a hereditary disorder. About 3000 people in Britain suffer from the disease at any one time. It usually begins after the age of 30 years. Early symptoms are twitching of limbs and muscles of the face. Mental symptoms other than dementia are common at first. As the illness progresses the movements become more marked and dementia occurs in most cases. There is now a genetic test but this is difficult for relatives who have to decide whether or not to have the test to see whether they may develop the disease. Some may wish to know and some may not.

Pick's disease is a rare form of dementia. It usually occurs between 50 and 60 years of age and in more women than men. Usually they have personality change followed by deterioration in memory and speech. The cause is unknown.

People with **Down's syndrome** often develop a dementia that is very similar to Alzheimer's disease, often in their 50s. Possible genetic links here have led to work on genetic links in other forms of Alzheimer's disease.

AIDS-related dementia is still being researched. Some people develop a slow onset type of illness, while others show rapid decline over a few months.

Repeated **head injury** is also associated with dementia. An example is the "punch drunk" syndrome seen in ex-boxers. Head injury is also thought to increase the likelihood of Alzheimer's disease.

"Reversible" dementias

Some conditions may look like dementia but are, at least in part, treatable. By some definitions these are not true dementias. **Sub-dural haematoma** is a blood clot due to bleeding on the brain surface usually caused by trauma. **Normal pressure hydrocephalus** occurs if something interferes with the usual circulation of the cerebrospinal fluid (the fluid in the spaces called ventricles in the brain). This may lead to dementia, walking difficulties and incontinence.

Alcohol can cause dementia – usually after prolonged heavy drinking. Some of this seems to be reversible if the drinker stops drinking altogether. In some people the memory is particularly badly affected compared to other abilities: this is called **Korsakoff syndrome**.

Hypothyroidism (lack of thyroid hormone) and **vitamin deficiency** can also look like dementia.

The person is still there

Whatever the cause of the dementia, and it can be difficult to determine the cause except at post mortem, each person has their own reality, drawn from past experience, relationships and personality. The condition fluctuates and even in severe dementia it is possible for attentive people to reach in from time to time, and for those who have a dementia to reach out and communicate in various ways.

The relationship between previous personality and physical and mental illness presents an ever-changing challenge to care staff, which must be met to ensure the preservation of dignity and maximum wellbeing of each individual.

Checklist for good practice

1. Not all old people are ill.
2. Old age itself is not an illness.
3. All illnesses, physical and mental, are more common with increasing age.
4. Remember that depression is common in people with or without dementia. It should be recognised and treated.
5. *Acute* confusion commonly points to a treatable condition and needs investigating.
6. Dementia is an illness which damages the person's ability to remember and communicate, but does not destroy the person.

CHAPTER 7

Promoting wellbeing, preventing abuse and inadequate care

Maria Scurfield

• Rights and respect • "Care" that was actually abuse • Who is at risk?
• How do we define and identify abuse • Procedures for reporting and discussion
• Preventing abuse and inadequate care – including strategies for
positive staff practice

Every older person, including and especially the person disabled by dementia, has rights, which include the following:

- the right to be valued as an individual
- the right to independence
- the right to privacy
- the right to choose
- the right to protection and safety
- the right to be consulted in decisions about their care
- the right of respect.

Abuse and inadequate care occurs when the older person is deprived of any of these rights.

"Care" that was abuse

Standards and expectations of dementia care have improved greatly over the past 10 years. Care practice should no longer be seen as task orientated with rigid routines or focused on physical care only. Those practices led to gross psychological neglect and inadequate care for people with dementia. The bad effects of such practices will include sensory deprivation, disorientation, withdrawal, hopelessness, helplessness, loss of identity, worsening of cognitive functioning and increased dependence.

We must all continue to challenge the attitude you are still very likely to meet – that the wellbeing of people with dementia is of little importance. From the other chapters of this book you will have seen that the wellbeing and quality of life of each person with dementia is of great importance, and the responsibility of all care staff.

Physical care is important but it is not enough; you need to care for the whole person. You should aim to enable each individual to make the fullest possible use of his or her abilities and to remain in touch with the world and other people.

Unfortunately for some older people, receiving care from others may lead to them being exploited, neglected and abused.

Who is at risk?

Older people who are vulnerable to abuse or inadequate care are most likely to be those who are dependent on others for their care. They may have physical, psychological, self-care and emotional difficulties; and may rely on another person to help them with a range of activities such as washing, dressing, feeding, mobility and toileting.

They may have special communication difficulties as a result of dementia or cerebrovascular disease, or may be suffering from visual and hearing problems, immobility, urinary or faecal incontinence. Another factor that makes abuse more likely is when the person has undergone a personality change or displays behavioural problems, which may occur in dementia, confusion or depression.

What is abuse?

It is not easy to define old age abuse and inadequate care. Some people do not believe that older people are abused, either in the community or in institutions. Another problem is that what one person sees as an abusive or neglectful situation may not be considered so by another.

For example, a nurse felt it was acceptable to keep a resident in a chair with a table across it for long periods of time because the resident wandered about and was at risk of falling. This is, however, clearly a form of abuse as it is used as a method for restraining the resident.

In order to simplify different definitions, abuse and inadequate care are defined in the box above.

What is abuse and inadequate care?

It is mistreatment of an older person which results in suffering and distress.

- **The abuse can be physical, psychological, financial or sexual.**

- **It can be a conscious and deliberate act, or it may be the inability of a carer to provide adequate care that meets the needs of the dependent person.**

- **Abuse and inadequate care can be a single incident, or part of a repeated pattern.**

Abuse and neglect can take place in a variety of environments where the older person is being cared for, including the person's own home, hospital wards, day hospitals, residential homes, nursing homes, day centres.

Different types of abuse

There are many different features of abuse and inadequate care:

- Physical abuse such as slapping, shaking, pushing, dragging, pulling hair, force feeding, restraining, misusing medication.

- Sexual abuse may include lack of privacy or dignity, insensitivity, unwelcome fondling, rape or buggering.

- Emotional and psychological abuse, which may include ridiculing, humiliating, blaming, intimidation, swearing, ignoring or frightening the person.

- Environmental abuse or neglect, which may include:
  – removing mobility aids, hearing aids and glasses;
  – withdrawing valued activities;
  – inadequate supervision;
  – not providing privacy or choice for the older person;
  – lack of stimulation;

– set rules and restrictions
  eg set bed times;
– deprivation of food, heat, clothing
  or comfort.

• Financial abuse, which may include withholding and misusing money, or theft.

The family carer

The role of the "informal" or family carer (see chapter 19) is both physically and mentally demanding. Usually an incident of abuse is brought on by a high degree of stress. Some carers find their role to be exhausting, frustrating and a seemingly endless commitment.

Studies indicate that there are some common factors for abuse and neglect by family carers. Awareness of these and help in resolving them may stop the abuse from occurring.

Factors making carers more likely to abuse include:

• when the person is totally dependent upon the carer

• when the carer has had to undergo considerable change in their personal and/or working life

• where there is a poor past or present relationship between the carer and the older person, particularly where there has been a reversal of the role between parent and child

• where the carer feels a sense of hopelessness and helplessness over their situation

• when the carer feels exploited and let down by health and social services

• when the carer finds specific tasks distasteful

• when the carer feels isolated, exhausted or stressed by the situation

• when the carer him/herself suffers physical or mental ill health.

Other factors include overcrowding; poor housing conditions with lack of privacy and personal space; history of abuse in the family; or the carer themself being abused by the dependent person.

The paid carer

Some of the factors for abuse and neglect by family carers could also be risk factors for paid carers. In addition, a consideration of factors known to have caused abuse and neglect in paid carers include:

• lack of training, support and supervision of staff

• low morale, partly due to low status attached to their work

• working in isolation from professional colleagues

• poor staff attitudes and behaviour

• having a "controlling" personality and behaviour

• poor staffing levels.

There may also be poor management practices which can include:

• no clear guidelines for staff about the philosophy, aims and objectives of care

• ineffective action when incidents occur

• failure to ensure standards of care are monitored.

Identifying abuse

There can be a number of reasons why older people with dementia do not report those who are abusing them, so all care staff should be vigilant for signs of abuse. A number of common indicators of abuse have been identified. However, it is very important not to use these indicators in isolation as a simple checklist. They should also not be confused with physical changes of the body associated with old age, or genuine accidents. The following lists have been identified in a number of research studies and reports:

Indicators of physical abuse

Frequent injuries and falls which are inadequately explained (injuries may include fractures or dislocations)
Bruises and finger marks in well protected areas, eg inside the arms and legs and "pepperpot" (knuckle marks) bruising to the chest
Unexplained cuts, lacerations and lash marks
Burns in unusual places
Excessive repeat prescriptions, or the underuse of medication
Bruising and/or bleeding in the genital area, and/or venereal disease.

Indicators of inadequate care

Poor nutrition
Weight loss
Dehydration
Hypothermia
Inappropriate and/or improper dress
An appearance of being unkempt, unwashed; poor hygiene
Unexplained fatigue (resulting from sleep deprivation)
Untreated medical problems
Avoidable pressure sores
Absence of glasses, hearing aids or mobility aids
Isolated in one room
Lack of stimulation.

Emotional and psychological indicators of abuse in the older person include:

Appears withdrawn or anxious and agitated
May seem afraid of the carer
May be more passive and withdrawn in front of the carer
Loss of motivation – may become depressed and/or unco-operative
Increase in level of confusion or disorientation
Increased levels of dependency.

Understanding who is at risk

The most important factor is your knowledge of and relationship with the older residents you are caring for. This, together with your knowledge of abuse and inadequate care, will help you understand who is at risk and how it can occur.

But it is also very important not to jump to conclusions when you encounter a situation that you may not feel comfortable about. Discussing this with a qualified member of staff will help you to concentrate your thoughts and feelings about what signs may be present, and relate these to your knowledge of what causes abuse.

Report and discuss

It is essential that you always report and discuss your suspicions and concerns about the residents and carers for whom you provide care, to a qualified member of staff as soon as possible.

When you have had the opportunity to discuss this, and you both feel confident that an abusing situation may be taking place, you will need to write this down. If you feel that a person is being abused by a colleague, or other paid or voluntary worker, this will need to be investigated by their manager.

There is no doubt that such an incident can be extremely traumatic for everyone involved in it. But you must not for one moment think that you should not report the incident in order to protect a colleague or a carer. You must at all times act to protect the vulnerable older person you care for.

In making your report, you should write clearly and accurately a description of the alleged abuse or inadequate care, including the name of the older person, the name of the alleged abuser and their relationship to the person. You should include the date and time of the incident and any signs you observed. In addition you may wish to list the factors present that are contributing to the situation.

It is important that you do not speculate about the abuse. Only write down the facts of what you have seen or heard. You may wish to add descriptions or suspicions of earlier incidents if any. You should give dates of these and any action taken then, and by whom.

It is important that you continue to provide care and support to the older person and their carer. This can be a difficult situation; but essentially, while not condoning any abuse or inadequate care, you should be prepared to continue to provide the same or an increased level of support where appropriate and while further investigations are being taken.

You may be asked to contribute to further investigations. Health and social services do have local policies and procedures to deal with these situations.

You may be asked to attend a disciplinary hearing or case conference which may also include the person, the carer, and the alleged abuser if it is not the carer. It is therefore important that you keep a copy of your original written report.

Preventing abuse and inadequate care

Much of what can be done to prevent abuse and inadequate care and promote wellbeing involves good practice in the care of older people with mental health needs, which is well described in the other chapters of this book. Care should provide the person with dementia with choices, privacy, stimulation and interests. You should encourage each person to remain as active and independent as possible and enable them to maintain social contacts. You should put yourself in

their shoes and reflect on the care you would want to receive for yourself in a similar situation. The care you provide for the residents should be of the same quality you would expect for yourself.

It is important to recognise that each member of staff is unique, in that they all have different coping mechanisms. Research has indicated that working with people who are demanding, have challenging behaviour or communication difficulties, can cause stress and "burn out" in staff. It is very important that staff are encouraged to talk about their feelings, and that they are supervised and supported at work. There are recognised support structures to achieve this, such as those described below.

Strategies to promote a positive staff framework for practice include:

• The key worker role, a named member of staff who is responsible for the continued assessment and care planning of individual residents. Care workers can also be assigned to a key worker. This enables more in-depth knowledge of the resident and their carers and provides them with choices about their care.

• Structured clinical and personal supervision sessions for each member of staff. These may include examining skills in responding to challenging behaviour.

• Regular meetings to discuss, plan and evaluate individual and group activities. This should include knowledge of individuals past lifestyle, interests, social activities and strengths. You may also wish to include carers and friends.

• Structured staff appraisal which allows a two-way review process of your work. This should include an acknowledgement of your strengths, achievements, weaknesses and needs.

• A developmental plan should be agreed

to focus on areas of weaknesses and build upon strengths.

• Planned induction programmes and ongoing training and development opportunities.

• Involvement in team meetings to constantly review the ward's philosophy, aims values and objectives.

• Improvements of clinical practices should also be discussed.

• Involvement in quality assurance programmes and standard settings to improve quality of care. One such method is Dementia Care Mapping (see chapter 20) which makes a detailed and objective evaluation of the care given to people with dementia in formal settings.

Checklist for good practice

1. Every person with dementia has rights. Abuse and inadequate care occurs when a person is deprived of any rights.
2. The wellbeing and quality of life of each person with dementia is the responsibility of all care staff.
3. You need to enable each individual to make the fullest possible use of his or her abilities and to remain a social being.
4. People who are abused or who receive inadequate care are likely to be those who are dependent on others for their physical and psychological care.
5. Always report and discuss your suspicions and concerns about a resident and carer to a qualified member of staff as soon as possible.

Resources

Kitwood T, Bredin K (1992) *Person to person: a guide to the care of those with failing mental powers.* Gale Centre Publications, Essex.

Pritchard J (1995) *The abuse of older people: training manual for detection and prevention.* Jessica Kingsley Publications, London.

Royal College of Nursing (1996) *Combating abuse and neglect of older people. Guidelines for nurses.* Royal College of Nursing, London.

Social Services Inspectorate (1993) *No longer afraid: the safeguard of older people in domestic settings.* HMSO, London.

Action on Elder Abuse, Age Concern England, Astral House, 1268 London Road, London SW16 4ER. Tel 0181 764 7648. Helpline 0800 731 4141.

CHAPTER 8

Activity and community involvement

Michael Broughton and Alison Johnson

• The normal activity of daily life • Helping everyone to feel they have a valued contribution to make • Household tasks • The world of work • Leisure and sporting activities • The wider community • Activities that involve the senses

Activities in daily life begin from the moment you get out of bed. While it is good to have a programme to occupy residents during the day, it is even more important that care staff look at how they can involve residents in the normal activities of daily life right through the day, from getting up in the morning to returning to bed at night.

For example, can they be encouraged to help make the bed, fluff up the pillows or draw back the curtains? Can they lay the table, clear away the crockery or help wash up? Simple tasks like these encourage conversation, help to maintain manual skills, and create a feeling of satisfaction in a job well done.

But most important of all, this sort of activity gives a continuing sense of role and purpose. How much better and more normal it is to go into the living room of a home and see some residents helping with meal preparation, others folding clothes ready to be aired, others looking at the paper or knitting – rather than seeing them sitting in a circle "doing an activity".

Why should we encourage activities? We need to be quite clear that we are not encouraging our residents to be involved in activity simply as a means of passing the time – or of saving on staff time. Indeed we may well need more staff if we develop activities suited to each individual's needs.

We encourage activities:
• to enable our residents to continue to lead as normal a life as possible and as much like their life was before they came to our home
• to stimulate residents' minds and bodies and bring them to the end of the day with a sense of achievement and satisfaction
• to help our residents feel valued and that they have a contribution to make.

On the other hand we must respect the rights of our residents to say "no" or to choose to sit and watch what is going on rather than join in. We have already seen that, in caring for people with dementia, the key thing to remember is that each person with dementia is an individual with dementia and that what we do with one resident is not going to work for all. Indeed an activity that Mrs Jones enjoys on Monday may be a complete failure on Tuesday, but may give her enormous satisfaction on Wednesday. So often we hear people saying "I tried that with Mrs

Jones and she wasn't interested" – but everyone has days when they feel like a particular activity or outing and other days when it is the last thing in the world that they want to do.

In considering activities, therefore, we need to find out what each individual likes doing, what they used to do in their earlier life and how we can involve them in the life and activity of the home to ensure that they continue to feel they have a role to play. A good home will be one where residents, staff, relatives and members of the community together live life to the full in, as far as possible, exactly the same way that we all live out our lives. We shall therefore look at activity under the broad headings that any one of us might use to review our daily, weekly or annual activities.

Activities related to household tasks

We are all, to a greater or lesser extent, involved throughout our lives in basic household tasks such as cooking, washing, cleaning, gardening and DIY. There is no reason why our residents should not continue to participate in these activities, if they choose to do so.

Cooking
Many homes in Australia, and some in this country, have made the kitchen the focal point of homes for people with dementia. The sights and smells of kitchen activities are a powerful reminder of home, and many residents are able to help with preparing food; for example peeling vegetables, making drinks or choosing their own jam to spread on a scone. Baking cakes is a popular activity and includes numerous opportunities for remembering recipes, the touch and smell of different ingredients and the pleasure of homemade food. A social event or

normal afternoon tea can provide the perfect excuse to enjoy the results.

Other residents like to help lay the tables or wash up, and involvement in the routine of mealtimes gives shape and form to the day – much more so than the unexpected arrival of a trolley from a distant and remote kitchen.

In one home, the residents were involved in every stage of making plum jam. First they went out in the home minibus to the orchard where they helped pick the plums. Back home, animated discussion followed, drawing on many years' experience of jam making. Residents discussed with staff ways of removing stones, of preparing the fruit and sugar, of sterilising the jars and testing for setting point. Argument followed over whether to cover at once or when cool and all the jars were labelled and stored. The following week the jam was sold at the monthly coffee morning and the residents were proud of their product and the contribution they were making to the amenity fund.

Cleaning
Many of our residents were accustomed to spending their mornings cleaning and polishing their homes. A film set in a dementia ward in a hospital showed a lady constantly running her hands along the window sills. Giving her a duster turned a "strange behaviour" into meaningful activity. Many residents would be happy to help in the daily routines of cleaning.

Laundry
This is another activity of daily living that, especially in the days before washing machines, filled a housewife's week. Why make laundry a distant activity for special staff in a special area? Many residents enjoy helping loading the washing machine, pegging out clothes and folding washing ready for ironing or airing.

Gardening

For some, gardening is a household task, for others a hobby or leisure activity. Living in a home need not mean an end to the pleasure of gardening. Raised flower beds may be helpful for residents with problems of mobility, but planting seedlings and bulbs can be done at a table.

Other people will find pruning or weeding rewarding activities and everyone will enjoy looking at plants and flowers in a well developed garden or border. Stimulating people's senses with the colour, smell and feel of natural, growing things will bring smiles, comfort and warmth. Seedlings, grown with care, can be sold at coffee mornings, like the jam, and bring satisfaction to their growers.

Sometimes over-enthusiastic gardeners dig up plants as well as weeds! However, a sign of a good home is one where staff patiently overcome such problems rather than planting prickly shrubs. A garden shed and outside toilet make gardening an even greater pleasure.

DIY

Many residents, especially the men, have spent weekends or evenings pottering about doing maintenance tasks about their home. Often staff can involve interested residents in shopping in a DIY store and helping with changing a washer, putting up pictures or other daily maintenance jobs.

The world of work

Many residents, male and female, have spent the greater part of their lives in the world of work, and since often through their dementia they are living in earlier years, it is very important for us to know the nature of their former work. In this area we can again often interpret their so-called "problem behaviours" by understanding what they are trying to tell us.

In one home, an old gentleman was always restless during the afternoon, and if given the chance would go into the office, pull envelopes out of the desk and place them in piles. He had worked in the sorting department of the local Post Office and an imaginative staff member provided him with bundles of envelopes which he was happy to sort in his "office" (or bedroom) every afternoon.

Herbie, an Australian engineer, was forever hovering round the boiler room until he was supplied with an engine in the courtyard and a set of tools. Mr Evans, a Methodist minister, was at first unwilling to agree to any visitors to his room, but was quite happy once he had a diary so that, as he had done all his life, he could consult the diary to ensure that he was free.

Another home, built for members of the printing trade, found enormous benefit from the showing of a work-related video of a newspaper works which encouraged reminiscence and conversation and a happy return to the years of work in the industry.

Leisure and sports

Too often this is the only area of activity which finds a place in care homes. But who spends all their days in leisure or sporting activity? Staff must appreciate that many people have no interest in arts and crafts, board games or carpet bowls. There is no reason why simply because someone has dementia they change the likes and dislikes of a lifetime. It is also important to realise that watching can be as important as participating; after all, many of our residents enjoyed watching sport on a Saturday afternoon, going on a social outing on Saturday night and spending a lazy Sunday afternoon with the family.

However, there are many who do enjoy these activities, and others who take up new activities in old age. Some examples are given below, but the possibilities are endless and depend very much on the individual likes and dislikes of residents – and of staff and volunteers, for the most successful activities are those where the joy and satisfaction are shared by residents and helpers alike.

Reminiscence

In a good home, each resident has his or her own life story book or memory box where items of particular significance are pasted or stored. Looking with a resident through these books or photographs often releases a fund of memories as do videos of past events. Old magazines, or videos of films from the 1930s, 1940s or 1950s are often more enjoyable for residents than modern films. Some homes take videos and photographs of outings and special events like birthdays so that they can be recalled later.

Quizzes on local knowledge, special interest subjects and 20th century history can be great fun and will give residents the chance to think, reflect, recall and share experiences. Never underestimate the mental ability of someone with dementia - you may be surprised at the volume of knowledge revealed.

Music

Simple movement to music, gentle exercise and limb stretching helps to keep people fit and mobile. It may also stimulate memories, even encouraging an impromptu sing-along. In the pre-television age, a traditional family event would have been gathering round the piano, singing songs or hymns. It is amazing how even for those who appear to have lost most of their language, the sound of a tune, and the patterned and orderly sequence of verses, can trigger off accurate recall of the words of a familiar song.

Favourites from the past create a feeling of warmth and security and an atmosphere of shared happiness. Often a resident with dementia is able to lead such a sing-along from the piano – fingers seem to recall the patterns of a tune even when reading music is no longer possible.

Arts and crafts

Some residents will enjoy art and craft activities such as painting, needlework, knitting or collage making. Others will loathe the very idea and choose to opt out of any activity of this sort. Particular enjoyment for some comes from tactile crafts like working with clay or doing finger painting. Others see these as infantile activities. Staff need to find out from residents or their relatives the sort of craft that each individual used to enjoy doing, and then help and encourage them to continue. For some, taking up a completely new activity may be exciting and liberating; there are many examples of new artists in their eighties or nineties.

The pleasure and fulfilment from such activities cannot be underestimated. In one home a resident without dementia decided to help her friend rediscover the pleasures of knitting. Through patient and painstaking tuition, a small garment was completed to the delight not only of the resident but of her daughter who said, with tears in her eyes, that her mother had not been able to knit anything for ten years.

Table games

Again some love and others hate table games. Old favourites like dominoes, ludo or pontoon can be brought out as and when the interest is there. Sometimes concentration may dwindle and the game may not be played to the end, but this doesn't matter. On the other hand, it may stimulate and bring out natural competitive skills in some people. Even if the participants end up stacking the dominoes following a brief game, or counting the numbers, pleasure will have been gained.

Active games

Some residents enjoy playing snooker, darts or carpet bowls, or patting a balloon from person to person. Sometimes, but by no means always, these physical activities appeal particularly to the male residents who are generally in the minority. We must make sure we don't forget the men. Being part of a male environment has often been very important to them and they may well socialise differently when not in female company; this should be respected and encouraged. Perhaps some male volunteers or members of staff could occasionally organise a "men only" time to meet this need.

Reading

Our residents belong to the age when books and reading were important leisure activities. Don't forget the pleasures of reading aloud – poetry, parts of well-loved books, or newspapers, both national and local. Old magazines, postcards and birthday cards all prompt thoughts and feelings of past times.

The wider community

Our residents are, or should be, members of the local community just like anyone else. A good home enables the residents to go out and about in the community and welcomes members of the community into the home. This, of course, includes relatives and friends of residents but also volunteers, school children, and others who live in the neighbourhood.

Shopping, visiting the library and other outside events

Although some care homes have their own shop, run by either staff or volunteers, it is much better for residents to be accompanied to local shops where they can choose and purchase their own sweets, toiletries, birthday cards or other personal requirements.

If Mrs Smith has lived all her life in a small community she will be well known there. If she can still get to her old local shops, she will be recognised there and will in turn recognise and remember the reason for the visit – collecting her pension or paying for the papers. Both Mrs Smith and the member of staff or volunteer with her will benefit from the fresh air and exercise, the stimulation of new and varied experiences – and maybe a cup of tea in a café together before they return.

Most local councils now have mobile visiting library services but again it is even better to be accompanied to the local library. As well as books, residents can now usually borrow cassettes, videos and other items like jigsaws and games.

Residents often enjoy attending coffee mornings and other local social events; and at one home, they nearly all choose to attend the regular tea dance in the assembly rooms.

Involvement with local churches

Many of the current generation of residents had a strong rooting in the Christian faith which, even if lost in adulthood, is regained in old age. Some are members of other faith communities (see chapter 2). The co-operation and support of the church and its community can be very important, especially for Christian-based care homes. Wherever possible residents should be enabled to attend worship in the local church of their choice. However, many homes are fortunate to have regular services of worship within the home. This is of paramount importance to frail older people who wish to have continuing faith and spiritual guidance. Services have been specially developed for older people with dementia, using symbols to help them remember and respond, such as a crucifix, candles or lectern, as well as large print hymn books.

A quiet time for prayer and reflection can be a great help to confused residents, and it is amazing how the words at the start of a hymn or prayer can stimulate total recall.

If care staff feel they are able to do so, it is good to share individual moments with a resident if it seems appropriate – saying Grace at mealtimes, a prayer at night or holding a resident's hand during a sad moment of reflection. Older people were brought up in a society that placed a strong emphasis on religion and therefore they attach a greater meaning to faith and spirituality. During our later years we all tend to spend more time reflecting on our beliefs, on death and dying and about our purpose in life. It is good if staff can encourage residents to reflect and express these kind of thoughts.

Relatives, volunteers and the community within the home

Another measure of a good home is the degree to which relatives, residents and the wider community are involved within the home. Such people can lend support with individual activities, organise or join in special events and accompany residents on formal and informal outings. They bring into the home news of the local area, fresh ideas and suggestions and time and patience to devote to residents.

Most homes have social occasions where residents, staff, volunteers, families and friends can get together and enjoy themselves. An entertainer, an old time music hall or country and western group with perhaps a raffle and a fish and chip supper, generate an excellent atmosphere which all can enjoy. A special birthday or golden wedding celebration are other excuses for a social event and, on occasions, a fundraising occasion like a beetle drive, coffee evening or summer fete give the whole community a sense of fulfilment and working together.

A nearby primary school may provide a concert or nativity play and secondary pupils may offer music, drama or crafts. Women's groups may come for coffee mornings or support individual residents who have no local family or friends. A local pianist may come to play for a sing-along, or an artist to help with painting. Church groups may join in worship, fellowship or prayer and provide comfort for those who are bereaved.

If your residents receive lots of visitors, it is a good idea for there to be a notebook for each resident recording dates and times of visits and something about the conversation or activities which took place. In this way relatives and staff are aware of visits and can help the resident to remember and recall happy occasions.

Daily, weekly and seasonal activity

People with dementia generally have particular difficulty with time and thus activities which help to reinforce a sense of time of day or week or season of the year are very important.

Time of the day

We have already seen that helping in, or seeing and hearing, meal preparation and table laying helps cue in the times for meals. Often there is a time of day when individuals are at their most alert, and other occasions when they are sleepy. Care staff must be sensitive to these individual daily patterns and plan activities accordingly. It may suit you to take residents shopping at 2pm, but if that is

January	Burns Night
February	Pancake Day
March	Mothering Sunday
April	Grand National Easter
May	Maypole dancing Cup final
June	Ascot
July	Wimbledon
August	Summer holidays
September	Harvest thanksgiving
October	Halloween
November	Bonfire Night
December	Christmas

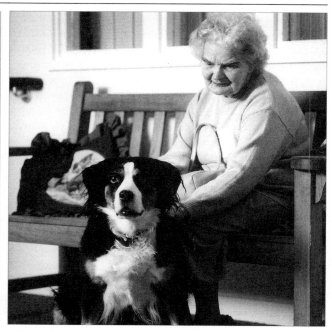

Left: Some ideas for special events through the year. Right: Many homes have a resident pet; the opportunities for touching, stroking and cuddling are appreciated by animal lovers.

when they like to have an afternoon sleep, it is not appropriate to disturb them, especially if they are as a result tired, awkward or grumpy.

Traditionally we all relax and begin to wind down before going to bed. People with dementia are no different and do not want staff rushing them and making them get ready for bed if they are comfortable in their chair.

Time of the week

Although it is not always possible for a home's weekly Church service to take place on a Sunday morning, it is not acceptable for the service to take place on whatever day and at whatever time suits the minister. Routine is important for us all; varied service times are bound to make residents feel disorientated. Similarly, it is better for a hairdressing appointment to occur at a regular time than whenever the resident can be fitted in.

Programmes on TV and radio may be important milestones in the week. Someone who has always watched *Neighbours* at lunchtime should be enabled to continue to do so. Likewise residents who have always watched football or like to watch *Songs of Praise* need to be reminded of the day and time to help them keep in touch.

Seasons of the year

The yearly cycle of special days and events provide us all with a framework for living and occasions to look forward to with anticipation. We can talk about them in advance, discuss similar festivals in the past and look back on the event with pleasure. Most homes make a special attempt to celebrate such events appropriately and often involve relatives, friends and volunteers in their planning and execution. Events might include those in the box above.

Involving the senses

Of course all the activities described in this chapter involve the senses, but there is a growing interest in massage, aromatherapy and other forms of sensory contact. These seem to by-pass the blocks to verbal communication that may have developed in the brains of people with dementia.

Some homes have found that using multi-sensory equipment has a relaxing, calming influence on people with dementia. Here the primary senses are stimulated by a unique combination of music, lighting effects, gentle vibration, tactile sensation and aromatherapy. A complete room can be expensive, but individual parts can be adapted for any home. The gentle lighting, smells, music, and tactile equipment create stimulation and communication and reduce agitation and anxiety in residents – and often in staff as well.

Many homes have found benefit from hydrotherapy provided that residents feel safe and supported in the pool. The warm water helps relaxation and the benefits often remain well after the session.

The presence of animals and the opportunities for touching, stroking or cuddling a pet dog or cat have proved valuable for some residents. Many homes have a resident dog or cat or encourage staff or visitors to bring in their pets. Some even allow residents to bring their own pets. While this at first sight seems appropriate since we ask residents to see the care home as their home, we nevertheless need to be aware of the problems of too many idiosyncratic pets - and the sensibilities of those who are allergic to or simply do not like animals.

At this point we should just mention the contentious issue of the role of soft toys and dolls for people with dementia. While some are concerned about infantilising and undermining the dignity of a resident who plays with a doll or teddy bear, others point to examples of adults with all their mental powers who take a bear to bed. For some people undoubtedly a soft toy is a perfect companion and helps to initiate conversation, and provide security and comfort. We must never dismiss any activity out of hand without looking carefully at its benefits to the resident.

Points to remember

1. As far as possible plan an individual programme for each resident, aiming to provide activity which will give them joy and stimulation and reflects past life styles, hobbies and interests. Activities of no interest could provoke "challenging behaviour".

2. See yourself doing things **with** residents, not **for** residents. Focus on ability, not disability.

3. Boost confidence; do not underline failure. Help your residents to live with their dementia, not feel that they are an inconvenience.

4. Focus on involvement, not achievement or quality of end product. It's the taking part that counts.

5. An activity organiser may provide ideas, but all staff should be involved.

6. Walk the residents' road, letting them lead the way and following their signposts.

7. Remember, just being with a resident is an activity in itself. Don't feel guilty that you are not busy "doing something".

8. Watchers may gain as much as participants. A resident who observes today, may decide to join in tomorrow.

CHAPTER 9

Mealtimes, eating and drinking

Tessa Perrin

• Mealtimes – a shared pleasure • Good nutrition in older age • Stimulating a poor appetite • Eating in company – the importance of the social setting • Maintaining independence • Help with feeding

No matter who we are, young or old, rich or poor, of this culture or that, food and drink play a vital part in our lives. Hunger and thirst are among the most basic drives we have; and our bodies' demands for the frequent and regular meeting of those needs mean that our lives are structured around food and drink almost from the moment we are born. The consistent daily pattern of two or three set mealtimes, and rather more drink and snack times, is a habit established early, and a routine that most people never change throughout their lives.

But fundamental as these events are to daily life and health, food is much more to us than satisfying drives, nourishing cells and providing a timetable to our day. The pleasure that we find in eating and drinking leads most of us to attach a major social significance to it. We centre most of our "coming together", whether as family or friends, around food and drink: the Sunday lunch, the coffee morning, the pub quiz night, the cricket tea.

A shared meal or a drink in a friendly atmosphere can promote communication and foster relationships in a strangely unique way – maybe it's something to do with sharing a pleasure together. And then perhaps because of these qualities, we give food and drink pride of place in our festivity and celebrations: the birthday cake, the wedding breakfast, the Christmas turkey, the champagne toast of achievement, the holy communion.

Only as we recognise the central place of food and drink in all our lives as individuals and members of communities will we appreciate the related needs of elderly people in our care. It is perhaps helpful to consider these needs from four perspectives:
• nutrition
• taste
• independence/dependence
• social setting.

Good nutrition in older age

People who keep to the principles of a well-balanced diet into old age are unlikely to suffer nutritional deficiency. Generally speaking, the type of diet that is appropriate for a younger person, is suitable also for the older person, although of course the physical process of ageing may mean that energy requirements are reduced. We do need to bear in mind however, that ill health, whether physical or psychological, can severely disrupt eating patterns, and therefore nutritional intake. So all care staff need a basic knowledge of good nutrition and how deficiencies can occur.

A diet containing a wide variety of foods is one of the best ways of ensuring adequate nourishment. Where possible, balanced portions of foods from the following groups should be eaten:
• proteins (meat, fish, beans) including dairy products (cheese, milk, eggs)
• cereals (bread, rice, pasta, breakfast cereals)
• fruit and vegetables, preferably fresh (but dried or tinned fruit/vegetables are good too).

In addition, six to eight cups of fluid per day is a vital part of a healthy diet.

If a person is generally well and comfortable, and neither losing nor gaining significant amounts of weight, you can be fairly sure that their diet is adequate. However, keeping a watch on weight is important: weight loss is not inevitable in dementia; it is much more likely to be a consequence of not getting enough food.

Finger foods (foods that can easily be eaten by hand) are useful for many people who have difficulty with cutlery. Both meals and snacks can be served in this way – even as portable "brown bag meals" for people who are unable to sit still at mealtimes.

Finger foods are served at room temperature so people can eat at their own pace. Spills are minimised so it can be easier to assess accurately the amount of food an individual has eaten. Direct physical involvement with the food may help to focus people's attention and encourage them to eat more.

However, to achieve an adequate nutritional intake from finger foods, extra snacks are needed throughout the day. Fibre and folate (normally obtained from breakfast cereals and green leafy vegetables) may be lacking, so the finger foods should include liver sausage, pâté or marmite, broccoli spears, orange, melon, green beans, wholemeal bread, muesli bars and cakes made with wholemeal flour.

Summarised from Eating Well for Older People with Dementia*.

Poor appetite

A common problem for older people is that reduced energy requirements lead to reduced food intake. A reduced food intake can in turn lead to a nutritional deficiency – a person is simply not getting enough of the required nutrients in the amount or the type of food that they are consuming. Nutritional deficiencies can affect people's physical and psychological health in all sorts of ways, including increased apathy and confusion, greater risk of infection, poor wound healing, skin problems and sores, muscle weakness and poor coordination.

If appetite is poor, care staff need to ensure that what is eaten is sufficiently nutritionally rich to accommodate bodily requirements. Smaller meals offered more frequently, snacks and finger foods (see box above) may be of assistance.

If a person cannot cope with the traditional "meat and two veg" it doesn't matter; a cheese and tomato sandwich can be nutritionally as rich. If we have grown up with three cooked meals a

> • **Care staff should be able to offer food and drinks for residents and patients whenever required. Snacks and drinks – such as sandwiches, fresh fruit, biscuits, tea, milky drinks, fruit juices and water – should be available all day and during the night.**
>
> *From Eating well for Older People with Dementia**

day, we may need to shift our thinking a little here.

Colour and presentation are important too. The traditional "invalid" diet of steamed white fish and mashed potatoes might be nutritionally adequate and easily digested, but it is bland and unappetising. A little attention to colour and garnish can make all the difference in motivating the flagging appetite.

Where difficulties of chewing and/or swallowing are the cause of reduced intake, it may well be that you will require advice or assistance, ideally from a speech and language therapist. But even with a liquid or semi-solid diet, there are still plenty of possibilities: soups, scrambled eggs, milk puddings, custards, stewed fruit and fruit purees. It is quite possible too, to liquidise conventional meals; but if you do this, try as far as possible to process each food separately. There is nothing more unappealing than the glutinous grey/green product of chicken pie, potato and peas.

There are always going to be times in residential care, when through illness or disability a person is regularly failing to take in enough nutrients. On such occasions good use may be made of proprietary nutritional supplements such as Complan and Build-Up. These might be used between meals, or where necessary, as meal replacements.

When diet has been significantly reduced or altered, constipation and dehydration can be a problem. Above all, an adequate fluid intake must be ensured. You can do this by presenting drinks in a variety of different ways – as tea and coffee, thin soups and milky drinks, fruit juice and squashes.

Constipation should be controlled by diet as far as possible. Wholegrain bread and cereals, wholemeal breads, pasta and brown rice, pulses (beans and lentils), vegetables and dried fruits are all good sources of dietary fibre, which provide bulk and assist the passage of food through the gut. Small amounts of pure bran can be added to soups, stews and gravies. Laxatives should be a last resort, and are rarely required where the diet is wholesome and fibre-rich.

Taste

Matters of taste are of course completely individual, and for this reason we need to get to know each person's own special likes and dislikes as well as we can. This may not be an easy task. The person with an advancing dementia may be unable to express their preferences and choices, and where this is the case we will need to consult with their relatives and friends.

There are occasions of course, where there is no one to ask, and here we are thrown back largely on trial and error, and our own observation. Where language has disappeared, non-verbal communication is often still quite intact. We need to be alert to expressions of taste and distaste and choice, which may be expressed through facial expression, vocalisation and gesture.

An appreciation of a person's culture

is perhaps a useful starting point in discovering taste. Knowing whether the person is Asian or Jewish, from the north of England or the south of Ireland, should give us a basis on which we can build up a picture of an individual's preferences.

We should be offering choices of menu to our residents from which they, or we on their behalf, can select each day. They should not, as is sometimes the case, have to select today what they will eat tomorrow. As far as is possible within the constraints of institutional life, residents should be free to have a drink or a small snack of their choice whenever they wish.

Sad as it is to say, care settings still exist where every resident gets half a beaker of milky, sweetened tea at set times only throughout the day. This is not individualised care. Maybe remembering how we feel when that friend doesn't manage to make our own tea or coffee quite as we like it, will help us to get it right.

We need, too, to try and accommodate those individual preferences that have been a matter of life-long routine or tradition: Bert's half of bitter before lunch every day, Freda's hot milk and digestives before bed, David's packet of Polo mints always kept in his jacket pocket. These things are the stuff of truly person-centred care.

Changes with age

Of the six senses, taste is the one that appears to have received least attention from researchers, perhaps because it is not crucial for independence and communication. Studies that have been carried out, however, indicate fairly clear changes to taste perception in ageing, losses of up to 50 per cent being reported in some people over 60 years

of age. This seems to be due mainly to a decline in the number of taste buds, and a reduction in flow of saliva.

However, actual decline in individuals is something most of us will never be able to measure, except by taking note of what our clients say. So it seems a good general principle of care to apply the same principles to the stimulation of taste, as we might to the other senses. Where we use bold, colourful and varied stimuli to make the maximum impact on vision, hearing, touch and smell, so we might use them for taste. We need to ensure that we offer hot and cold, sweet and savoury, bland and spicy, heavy and light, crunchy and smooth. With such a large range of foodstuffs and beverages available to us today, we have an enormously diverse resource on which to draw for stimulation. Let us make use of it.

Social setting

Mealtimes are above all things opportunities for socialisation. There are of course some people who prefer to eat alone; indeed there are times when all of us like to eat undisturbed, in peace and quiet. But generally speaking most of us enjoy the shared pleasure of eating in company.

Dementia is an isolating condition, in which a person's avenues of communication are progressively impaired; relationship is fractured, interaction disrupted and the person becomes more and more cut off from the social network around him, increasingly enclosed in a world which we do not yet understand. We can use the familiarity of mealtimes to work against that isolation. A few pointers may help:

• It hardly needs saying that the dining-room environment is important. We all know the difference between an evening at a comfortable restaurant, and lunch at a motorway cafe on Bank Holiday Monday. Thinking about why one is more pleasant than the other should give us some indicators. The touches which make all the difference are often quite simple things; a prepared table setting, maybe flowers; tables accommodating a small number of people and a spacious setting – privacy within company; courteous service; soft music.

• There should be some flexibility regarding mealtimes. Most institutional settings have to conform to certain set mealtimes, and certainly with regard to the main cooked meal of the day, this is not unreasonable. But there is no reason why breakfasts and snack meals should not be made available as required. Our task is to sustain as far as possible each individual's preferred routine. If that has always meant breakfast at 6.00am for one person and at 10.00am for another, so be it. It might not fit our tidy routine, but it is person-centred care.

• Although it may not be possible in some units, we should consider making provision for our clients to eat with their relatives and friends in private on odd occasions, perhaps at times of celebration, or of special need. Not all will want to make use of such a facility, but some families will value immensely the opportunity for such shared privacy.

• Although it is still far from common, some unit staff have adopted the practice of sharing their mealtimes with residents (those staff will then need to take a break at another time). This does help in breaking down the "us and them" barrier. Why should we eat in separate places at different times? In addition, sharing mealtimes enables staff to assist the more dependent person in an unobtrusive way, and to keep a consistent check on quality control – quality of food, of service, of setting.

• From time to time, we are likely to have a resident whose disturbed behaviour is not tolerated by other members of the unit. This might be due to noise, shouting or screaming, or possibly to unpleasant or messy eating habits.

This is a difficult problem, often not easily resolved. There are occasions when we have to remove such a resident from the main dining group, sometimes for their own safety, sometimes for the wellbeing of other residents. We do not wish to penalise a resident for something which is most likely a feature of their dementia and their institutionalisation, so we need to be a little creative in our handling of such a matter.

Perhaps we need to think around removing the resident concerned to a different part of the dining area. If the problem is noise, could the resident share a table with those who have the most profound hearing impairment? If it is messy eating, could they share with other messy eaters? If the problem is interfering with others, could the resident sit at a small table just a little apart from the other tables?

Another alternative is to have a completely separate dining room for those who have mealtime difficulties, where there is some privacy, and perhaps an increased staffing allocation. There are no easy answers; each problem is quite individual and needs to be addressed as such, but we do need to bear in mind that forcing someone to eat on their own is not an option.

It is likely that most units which care for people with dementia will have a resident group with a wide range of ability between them. Some will be quite independent at the meal table; others will need assistance with all aspects of eating and drinking. And, as the course of dementia progresses, most people will demonstrate some decline in ability. Our main task is to find a sensitive balance between encouraging a resident to retain the independence they have, and recognising that certain skills have gone for good and require assistance. Finding the right approach is generally a matter of knowing the resident well, and coming to a team decision about how much help is needed.

Independence

For the person who needs to retain some independence, there is of course, a wide variety of mealtime aids. Your local branch of Boots the Chemist will have a catalogue of all the most popular and useful pieces of equipment. More often than not, all that is required is a non-slip mat and a plate guard to offer some stability, but the range is vast and can include some very sophisticated equipment.

It is useful to get to know about the more common items. A plate warmer is a thoughtful addition to the place setting for the slow eater. Cutlery with large, padded or moulded handles can mean independent eating for the person with arthritic hands. There are many possibilities. If you are in doubt, request an assessment from your local occupational therapist.

Before we bring in the equipment however, we need to have made some very basic checks on the residents first. Are they wearing their glasses? Have they their dentures in? Are the dentures well-fitting? How is the person sit-

ting? If they are slumped in an armchair they will not find it easy to eat independently – much better to sit close to the table in an upright chair.

You may also need to think through the matter of fingers: what of the resident who can't or won't use cutlery and prefers to eat with fingers? For some care staff, this goes against the grain of social taboo: it doesn't happen in polite society, it is demeaning and degrading. Well, person-centred care demands that our clients dictate the style of their care as far as possible; if roast beef, vegetables and gravy eaten with fingers means independence, choice, self-determination and tactile stimulation for our client, we have no grounds for arguing against that.

Is it better to be the passive recipient of food from a spoon by a stranger, than actively to assert our ability, individuality and preference, even if rather messily with fingers? This is a question we need to answer, for we will all meet it sooner or later.

Dependence

There comes a time for many people with dementia when their self care skills are so diminished that dependence is inevitable. It is still possible to retain dignity at mealtimes, even for the most severely impaired person. But this does require skilful and sensitive handling from staff. If your client is reaching that stage of dementia and disability which has been called the vegetative state, and requires maximum assistance, there are a number of things to bear in mind:

• Lift and support the person into a sitting position to eat. Many severely impaired residents spend their days in recliner chairs. They must be moved to an upright position in order to chew, swallow and digest efficiently.

• Some kind of protector for clothes is usually required. This is not particularly desirable, but it is a lot more dignified than shirts and dresses encrusted with the remains of the last meal, and considerably less time- and effort-consuming than repeated changes of clothes. There is a variety of disposables to choose from, which are quickly and easily removed as soon as the meal is over.

• Sit close to the person you are feeding and give them your attention. Use their name frequently and tell them what you are offering them. Warn them as each mouthful approaches; a verbal reminder, or a light touch of the lips with the cup or spoon is usually sufficient to engage the feeding reflex. (Speech therapists can give expert help with swallowing problems.)

• Watch closely for signs of pleasure or distaste: the change in facial expression, the gesture, the refusal of food. Be prepared to change the meal to an alternative if you think that your client does not like it.

• Above all talk to the person, even if only about inconsequential things. It doesn't matter if they don't respond; we never know how much they can hear. Talk about what is happening on the unit; talk about yourself, your family. You are all that is left for the client of the social setting, the shared pleasure of mealtimes. Try to make the most of that.

Mealtimes can often be perceived as a chore by staff in dementia care units. They are certainly hard work. But for our residents, they are the focal point of the day. Indeed, for some residents they are the only events of the day in which they actively engage. Commonplace as they might seem to us, they are for

many the high points in an otherwise passive and listless routine.

Care staff have an immense, easily available resource at our fingertips, which we might use for enriching and enhancing the impoverished lives of those elderly persons in our care. Food and drink are always familiar, always welcome. Let us learn how to use them to their maximum effect.

Checklist for good practice

1. People with dementia need time. Never rush mealtimes. Think 'finger foods'.
2. Do your best to find out a person's lifelong food habits and tastes.
3. Become an observer of responses to food. Even people without speech can usually find some non-verbal way of expressing choice.
4. Don't be bound by tradition. If somebody wants a cake sandwich, there is nothing wrong with that.
5. Plan the mealtime social setting together as a staff team. Everyone's contribution and point of view is valid in this important task.
6. Come to a team decision about messy eating. This often upsets relatives and visitors, and you need to be able to state your case with confidence.
7. If we can think of food as a therapeutic resource rather than just a biological necessity, good practice is bound to follow.

Resources
Eating Well for Older People with Dementia: a good practice guide for residential and nursing homes and others involved in caring for older people with dementia. Report of an expert working group (1998) published by VOICES (Voluntary Organisations Involved in Caring in the Elderly Sector). Available from PO Box 5, Manchester M60 3GE. Credit card orders: 0870 608 0213.

CHAPTER 10

Encouraging movement and mobility

Tracy Packer

- *Are you really encouraging independence and promoting mobility?*
- *What can affect or restrict movement* • *The little things that matter a lot*
- *Good communication* • *The effects of the environment* • *Safe manual handling*
- *When just a little help is needed* • *Pressure area care*

Sometimes I can walk into an area of care and very quickly assess how much independence is encouraged and whether as much mobility as possible is promoted. Time and time again, I see a person with dementia sitting forward in his chair just attempting to stand up, only to be pushed back into the chair by a well meaning care worker saying:

"Sit down Bob! You can't get up now, there'll be a nice cup of tea along in a minute."

A similar variation on this theme often takes place. Bob has, after a huge effort, successfully managed to stand up and shakily walked a few yards up the corridor. He is again taken by the hands and led back to his chair, often being scolded: "You can't go there Bob, now just sit down for a little while will you?"

Zimmer frames and walking sticks are carefully "tidied away" out of arms' reach, and small tables are firmly positioned in front of people sitting passively in their armchairs. Does this happen purely out of a need to keep an area clutter-free, or to ensure that food and drink can be reached? Or is there, in fact, an insidious kind or restraint taking place?

There is much that care workers can do to limit or encourage the amount of movement a person can be enabled to achieve. Promoting optimum mobility involves a certain amount of risk-taking, but the likely improvement to a person's quality of life always makes it worthwhile.

Promoting mobility

Many people with dementia will never have difficulties getting around, but some people do experience severe problems in this area. Mobility can be affected when people get further medical problems as a result of, or as well as, the effects of their dementia. They may also be affected as a direct result of damage to the parts of the brain which co-ordinate movement and balance.

Conditions which might affect mobility

- Conditions causing pain in the joints and muscles, particularly finger, hip and knee joints, may restrict a person's ability to get around. These may be arthritis, rheumatism, gout or bone fractures.

- Diseases which affect the circulation can also affect movement. Long-standing diabetes may lead to a dulling of sensations in the fingers and toes. Heart problems and high or low blood pressure can lead to dizziness and fainting, particularly after lying down and getting up too quickly.

• Migraine can severely affect vision and perception, and tinnitus (ringing in the ears) can affect the mechanism in the inner ear which co-ordinates the ability to balance.

• Some drugs can make people drowsy, unco-ordinated and unsteady. Alcohol alone can also do this, but even small amounts of alcohol mixed with some medication can have the same effect.

• Sometimes the ability of the brain to make sense of distance and space, as well as tell the difference between patterns, shadows and objects, can be severely affected by damaged eyesight or even the dementing process. This may make a person feel too frightened to move, or may contribute to unsteadiness or accidents which do not appear to have an obvious cause.

• Chest conditions such as asthma, bronchitis, infections and lung cancer can render a person too breathless to make even the smallest movements or shortest walks bearable. Anaemia may also make someone breathless.

• Any condition which weakens muscles and bones, may lead to a restriction of the ability to bend, stretch or support one's own body weight. Nutritional deficiencies, damaged tendons/ligaments, and obesity are just a few of these.

Encouraging independence

Often, when we know that someone can walk with only minimal assistance, it is easy to fall into the trap of thinking that they are being lazy or stubborn when they refuse to change position or walk anywhere. The other trap is, of course, to blame the process of dementia. This is easily done, and when a person with dementia refuses to "come for a little walk", you may hear comments like:

"Oh don't worry about what he says, he's very confused and doesn't know what's going on. Just do it anyway."

This kind of scenario can lead to great frustration for everyone. It is often the result of care workers automatically "blaming" the dementing process for a person's behaviour, instead of accepting that there might be perfectly good reasons why they should **not** do what you have asked them to do. The difficulty is in finding out what these reasons are, and doing something about them. In an ideal world these reasons should be discovered before a "job" needs to be started. But this is often easier said than done!

Consider the simple things in life
Some ladies are unhappy about going anywhere without their handbags. If they are unable to manage their bag as well as a zimmer frame, there are special net bags which can safely be attached to the frame to hold handbags etc. This may seem a trivial detail to you, but the walk will be much more enjoyable if you take such concerns seriously.

Some people may be afraid of losing a comfortable seat in their absence. Others may be afraid of their trousers or underwear falling down. Be sure that belts and braces are well fastened, buttons are done up, catheter bags have been drained, and that they and other continence aids are discreetly hidden.

Has the person you are about to walk with been to the toilet recently?
Many people live in fear of having an "accident" in front of everybody when they are walking. It is often worth dis-

creetly offering to take them to the toilet before you start. This can of course be part of getting them moving. Other people may have a urinary infection, or stress incontinence which makes them feel as if they need to be very close to a toilet at all times. Even if they have appropriate continence aids, and lots of reassurance, you may have to compromise with a circular walk in the general area.

So that you can chat while walking with them, ensure they are wearing hearing appliances if they use them, as well as dentures and spectacles. Zimmer frames and walking sticks often get mixed up, so ensure they are labelled or easily identifiable. Always make sure they are used.

What is the routine in your area?
Some people may think they will miss out on a cup of tea, their mealtime, or even a visitor, if they go for a walk at a specific time. Emphasise that they will be back on time and make sure that they are.

If they have missed out on a drink, make sure you get one for them on their return. If you do not, they may refuse to come with you in future.

Try to have a chair ready at the end of the walk. Some people will refuse such a journey ever again, because they had to stand in front of a room full of people staring at them while a chair was being found.

Imagine how you might feel walking into a room full of strangers, without having a chair to sit on when you get there: then having to stand there feeling like a trouble maker, or the odd one out, while another chair is being found?

Don't forget the less obvious things
Bunions, corns, callouses, verrucae and ingrowing toenails may seem common to you, but they are serious enough to hinder any active mobility. Make sure a referral to a chiropodist is made in order to

sort these out. This should be done as soon as they are noticed, and long before intensive rehabilitation begins.

Not long ago, an unfortunate chiropodist I knew was kicked in the face by a very frightened lady who was having her feet done after a hip operation. The nursing staff had neglected to give her any pain killers! Chiropodists can't do their job properly if this is neglected, and such an oversight will only delay a person's recovery. If you think someone is in pain, let a trained member of staff know about it immediately.

Ill fitting shoes and loose, insecure footwear can all hinder movement. So can pain from arthritis, gout, leg ulcers and many other medical conditions. A headache can be all it takes.

Get to know the person, and the signs they show when they have pain. They may not always be able to tell you about it, or even point to the place where there is pain. However, they may become withdrawn, fidgety or even "guard" the area that is in pain. The more you know, the better equipped you will be to do something about it.

Have you allowed enough time?
In the world of health care, many of us would dearly love to have more time. However, all too often we inflict the everyday busyness of our daily routines upon the people with dementia in our care. I'll give you an example:

It was a very busy shift with all of the staff rushing to and fro trying to catch up with all the work that had yet to be completed. Mrs Smith was waiting for an ambulance to take her to an important appointment. It was late. She had sat there patiently waiting for almost an hour, when suddenly two burly men and two members of staff burst in through the door. One of the men said:

"I hope this won't take too long, as

we're already behind and we've got another three pick-ups to do yet."

The two nurses rushed to Mrs Smith's side. She was startled and her eyes widened as they took each of her arms and, without speaking to her, attempted to stand her up.

Mrs Smith was having none of it. She dug her heels down, and pushed her bottom deep into the back of her chair. By this time she was very frightened and refused to go anywhere. It took all four of them half an hour to persuade her to get into the ambulance. You can imagine what state of mind she was in by the time she reached her destination. How would you like to have been the care worker at the other end, looking after Mrs Smith when she arrived?

If only someone had had the foresight to spend just five minutes with Mrs Smith as the ambulance arrived, explaining what was about to happen. It would have saved everyone a lot of time and unnecessary distress.

Are you making yourself clearly understood?

It obviously helps if a person understands what it is you are doing, and what it is you want them to do. We take so much of the spoken word for granted, but it is very important to be clear and concise. Simple words, short sentences, and plenty of repetition can often make life for everyone a whole lot easier (see also chapter 3). It is also important to watch carefully and listen, so we don't misunderstand.

If you had a very poor memory, what would you make of this: "Right, Mr Jones, I'm just going to make sure your slippers are on properly, then if you could stand up for me, we can take a little walk to the dining room. Can you just put your hands on the arms of the chair and push up, then I'll be able to help you, OK?"

The chances are that Mr Jones is either still thinking about getting his slippers on at this point, or he's wondering what it is you're going to help him with. Either way, you can be pretty sure that no movement in any direction will have taken place. This is a better approach:

"Hello Mr Jones. It's lunchtime." (Pause.)

"Would you like to come to the dining room with me?" (Wait for his response.)

"I'll just check your slippers." (Do this.)

"Are you ready to go to the dining room?" (Await response.)

"I'll help you." (Offer him your arm.)

"Now get a good grip on the arm of the chair." (Guide his hands if necessary.)

"Good. Now push yourself up." (Wait for this to happen, and repeat the instruction if necessary.)

"Are you all right?" (Check that he is.)

"The dining room's this way Mr Jones." (Point out the correct direction before starting to walk.)

"Well done." (Always offer praise and reassurance.)

What are your non-verbal cues saying?

The ability to understand words and language is very often damaged in people with dementia. This may mean that no matter how hard you try to keep things simple and to the point, there are sometimes great difficulties in making yourself understood. This can be frustrating for all concerned.

Always be aware that your body and face tell a "thousand stories" about what sort of mood you are in, how busy or interested you are, or what you think of somebody. People with dementia can become very good at understanding what we mean by observing our complex body language. We can turn this to our advantage by using gestures, mime, and often specific sounds, in order to make ourselves clear.

Edward refused to get out of bed for the first weeks after he was admitted to a specialist dementia unit. He would either get up around lunchtime, or the staff would attempt to wrestle with him to get him up sooner. It wasn't because he was tired and liked a lie in, which would have been fine, but he would point at the floor showing great fear and shaking his head.

The staff were baffled, but after one of them started some life story work with him, he found out that the gentleman was scared of water and had been involved in a nasty swimming accident when he was younger.

They then realised that the shadow cast on the shiny floor by the fine patterned curtains looked very "watery" as it moved about. When they closed the main curtains and put a light on when it was time to get up, there were no further problems.

When assisting someone to get up out of a chair, or walk, or sit back down again, it is important to give lots of reassurance in the form of smiles, nodding of your head, frequent eye contact, or thumbs up signs. A reassuring squeeze of the hand (or firm touch on the shoulder, if that's too personal) may just make the difference between someone giving up or successfully completing the task in hand.

Use your hands and eyes to indicate clear directions. Always try to appear calm, even if you are in a rush! Apply the same principles to non-verbal communications as spoken ones. That is: one instruction at a time, don't confuse your messages, and *listen*.

What effect does the environment have?

There is no doubt that the layout of a care setting can have a significant effect on the manner in which people with dementia can or cannot get around.

Floors that slope without warning can lead to a feeling of disturbed balance and uncertainty: people with dementia often slow down and grasp handrails more tightly if this happens. The change in texture from linoleum to carpet may affect the way wheels on a zimmer frame function, or the way the ground feels underfoot.

Pools of bright light or darkness across a corridor can be very deceptive, particularly if a person already has visual difficulties, as can heavy shadows and floor patterns. Strips of dark shadow or carpet edging can appear to be a step, and lead to a person refusing to go any further without any apparent reason.

Keep clutter and unnecessary objects out of the main thoroughfares in your area. If the place is turned into an obstacle course, you increase the chance of nasty accidents, "traffic jams" and general mayhem. Remember, if getting from A to B becomes a major chore, it is unlikely that someone will attempt it more than a very few times. Ensure that any spillage of fluids, talcum powder, food, etc, is cleared up immediately.

In many care environments, the most cluttered time of day is the morning, when hygiene needs are being met, beds made, and much of the general cleaning is taking place. At this time a plethora of linen skips, mops and sponges, buckets of water, cloths, detergent bottles, hoover/buffer leads, and the obligatory small pile of odds and ends from the floor which have been swept into a neat pile awaiting the bin, have to be negotiated.

It is important not to take these things for granted. If you can anticipate a problem, make sure you offer explanations and reassurance to the person well before they come across it. Ensure there are handrails along the way and that these are secured safely to the wall, free from splinters and clear of debris.

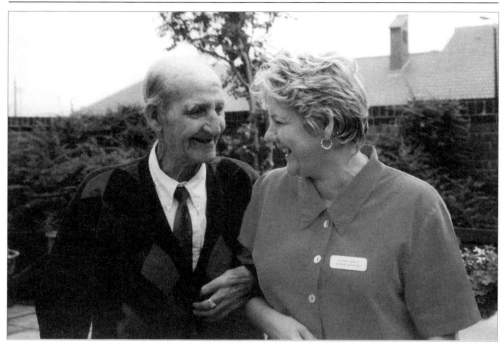

When assisting someone, reassurance and smiles help a lot. Try to appear calm, however busy you are.

Does the person actually want to do it?

Sometimes there are things we want to do that involve the person we are caring for. It is important that we don't get so carried away with a task that we don't offer the person a choice over what is happening. Sometimes a person will simply say "No". Other times they may not speak, but simply refuse to comply with what it is you want, and do their utmost to make it difficult to complete.

If you go ahead and make someone do something against their will, you will damage any trusting relationship you have been building up, and in the case of moving someone, you may even hurt yourself.

This is unnecessary. If you've considered some of the simple things that were mentioned earlier, and they still do not wish to comply, it is wise to respect a person's wishes. What is the worst thing that can happen? You can always come back

and try again later. People with dementia should be able to take some control over what is happening to them. If they are able to be assertive, consider it a complement. After all if they were too scared of you, they might have just complied and been very unhappy.

Are you confident in what you are trying to do?

Keep yourself up-to-date with the current manual handling regulations. You owe it to your colleagues and those in your care to do this, but most of all, you owe it to yourself.

Always use the equipment that is provided, and if you are not sure how it should be used, it is your responsibility to find out before attempting to use it. Most places allocate a member of staff who is responsible for updating everyone in manual handling skills and regulations. Find out who it is and use them – consult them and ask them to show you the best way to do things. If you do not have one, or do not know who it is, go to the person in charge and ask them about it.

People with dementia can often tell whether you know what you are doing or not. If there is any hint of uncertainty in what you are doing or how you are doing it, they will very often pick it up. How keen would you be to let someone lift you out of a bed or bath with a complicated-looking piece of machinery, if you suspected they did not really know what they were doing? If a person is frightened about this, they may not let you near them in the first instance. It is not surprising that if someone has had a traumatic experience with a poorly handled hoist before, they are unlikely to want to repeat the experience.

Safe manual handling

An estimated 40,000 care staff are off sick with back problems every year, and over 3,600 give up their work every year because of back injury. Do not become another one of these statistics. Take the law seriously; it exists to protect you.

There are three key issues to consider:

• Whenever possible, you should avoid manual handling which involves a risk of injury.

• If you cannot avoid it, a written assessment of the manual handling activity should be made by a trained member of staff. This should give detailed guidance on the way you should approach the load (person), the task in hand, the immediate environment and the abilities of the person undertaking the task.

• Every step should be taken to reduce the risk to the lowest possible level which is reasonably practicable. This means using mechanical aids as much as possible.

An increase in knowledge of safer han-

dling over the last few years has led to new guidelines on handling. This approach focuses on four main areas:

The task
How will the handling affect your body movement or posture? Will it involve:
– twisting the torso?
– stooping?
– stretching upwards?
– too much lifting or lowering?
– too much carrying?
– too much pushing or pulling?
– sudden movement of the person with dementia?
– frequent & prolonged physical effort?
– not enough rest and recovery?

The load
In the context of this chapter, the "load" refers to the person you are thinking of handling and/or moving. Is this person:
– heavy?
– bulky or awkward to hold?
– difficult to grasp?
– agitated or likely to move?

The environment
The conditions that you work in can have an important effect on your ability to work safely. Is there:
– plenty of room to use a good posture?
– uneven, slippery or unstable flooring?
– any variation in the floor level or work surfaces?
– too low or too high temperature or humidity?
– low or dazzling lighting?

The abilities of the individual
The more you know about your own capabilities, the easier and safer it will be for everyone concerned. Does the job:
– require lots of strength, or a particular height of person?
– create risks for those who might be pregnant or have a health problem?
– require special information or training?
– become more difficult because of protective equipment or personal clothing?

What this all means is that by carefully thinking about what you have to do, well before you have to do it, you can reduce the risks to yourself. The person can often help out considerably if you know what you are doing, and they understand what it is you want them to do. However, a proper assessment may indicate that the risks are simply too great, and mechanical assistance should be used.

Are you looking after your back?

There are many things you can do to protect yourself from painful and un-necessary back injuries. Remember it is important to be responsible to yourself and your colleagues. If you are not, you may suffer the consequences for the rest of your life.

The daily routine

Many of the things that care workers are involved with during their normal, daily routine can contribute towards a future back injury.

Consider how many of the things mentioned below are part of your daily routine. Then think about how many stretches, twists and bends you make to get that task completed. Finally, think about how you might change the way you do these jobs by working with other colleagues, sitting down, or using the equipment or adaptions that are provided.

• Making a bed by yourself

• Making a bed in a restricted space with little room to move

• Bending over a low bed while making it

• Leaning over a bed to reach something on the locker at the other side of it

• Stooping over a person while taking their blood pressure

• Reaching for an item on a shelf much higher than you

• Moving a heavy piece of furniture.

The following are not only bad practice but dangerous for your back too:

• Standing up or leaning across a table to feed someone

• Standing when talking at length to someone who is sitting

• Moving a static chair with a person in it.

Posture

If you have to lift at all, it is important that you are aware of the correct way to position yourself. The main aim is to avoid any movement which may lead to twisting, stretching or loss of balance. Seemingly trivial details such as tight, restrictive clothing and dainty footwear will contribute to bad positioning. Consider these points:

• Is this lift really necessary?

• Is there any equipment you should use instead?

• Is the area around you free of hazards?

• Do the patient and any colleagues you are lifting with, fully understand what will be done?

• Is there enough room for you to bend at the knees?

• Are your feet apart by a hip width to help maintain your balance?

• Is one foot facing the direction you are going in?

• Are you as close as possible to the person, to reduce potential back strain?

• Have you got a good, dependable hand-hold?

• Is your back straight?

• Are you really concentrating on the task to be done?

Mechanical aids

It is the responsibility of employers to provide suitable equipment for manual handling purposes. It is the careworker's responsibility to make sure they understand exactly how pieces of equipment work, and inform themselves in order to stay up to date. Read the manufacturer's information, attend manual handling update courses, and remain competent not ignorant! Above all, use the equipment you are provided with, do not consider "just managing" or "getting by" without it.

You must also report any damage or operational failure to the person in charge immediately. If equipment is not working, it should be taken out of use and clearly marked as damaged. Failure to do so could lead to other care workers and/or patients injuring themselves needlessly.

Accident forms

If you think you have pulled a muscle or hurt your back in any way during your working day, you must let the person in charge know about it, and you will need to fill in an accident form.

You have a responsibility to yourself, your colleagues and your residents, to refrain from any manual handling at all while you have discomfort. It may even be more appropriate for you to stay away from work.

Accident forms may seem like tedious paperwork, but they are there to protect you. They may also provide evidence on your behalf, particularly if you feel that your injury was a result of negligence by your employer. Always fill in an accident form.

When just a little help is needed

There are many people in our care who are never totally dependant on mechanical aids to get about. However, they may need some help to get out of their bed or chair. There is a fine balance between

assisting someone and actually lifting them, and it is important to understand the difference.

The following sequences of instructions, given one at a time by you, can help people retain the skills and muscle strength for independent movement .

Sitting down

Stand with your back facing the chair.
Put one foot a small distance behind the other.
Feel the edges of the chair with the back of the legs.
Lean down slightly from the hips, and grasp one or both of the arm-rests.
Lower your bottom right into the back of the chair.
Raise your shoulders until your back is straight.
Relax.

Moving to the front of the chair and standing up

Lean forward.
Hold arm-rests firmly.
Raise one buttock, and then the other to rock your body to the front of the chair.
Bring feet back towards the edge of the chair.
Place feet slightly apart, with one foot a little in front of the other.
Lean right forward, "face over feet".
Push up from arms and hands on the arm-rests, until your feet are able to support your weight.

Sitting further back in bed

Sit and lean forward.
Put both of your hands behind your buttocks.
Place them palm down on the bed.
Bring one knee up, keeping the base of your foot firmly down on the bed.
Move bottom back by pushing with your heel and hands.

**Getting up from the floor
(when there is no obvious injury).**
From flat on your back, aim to lie on your side.
Push up onto your hands and knees. The care worker should position a chair alongside.
Place hand nearest the chair, onto the seat or arm-rest.
Raise knee furthest from the chair, so that your foot is flat on the floor.
Push up with your hand and foot.
Get into position for sitting down.

Pressure area care

When skin and the area beneath it becomes damaged as a result of continuous unrelieved pressure, a person can develop what is known as a "pressure sore". These form when the blood supply to an area is cut off, and are more common on the lower buttocks, hips, heels and bony protrusions of the body.

Pressure sores are most often an unnecessary result of not taking movement and mobility seriously. They are painful wounds, which can be a source of infection, indignity, and disgust.

There are four main causes of pressure sores. These are:
Direct damage – A nasty fall, bump or graze disrupts the blood supply to an area, causing the surrounding tissue to die.
Shearing – The skin is dragged and grazed over a hard surface, causing small blood vessels to die. This can happen with poor manual handling techniques, or when heels and bottom slide down a bed.
Friction – This happens when parts of the body rub each other. Areas under the breasts, between the thighs and under-folds of skin are most vulnerable. Sweating or dampness following bathing

can make the problem worse. These sores feel like burns to the person who has them.
Compression – Tissue that is squashed between bone and a hard bed or chair for more than two hours will begin to have a damaged blood supply. This can lead to a pressure sore.

Preventing pressure sores.
It is important that care workers take responsibility for identifying risk factors that can contribute to the formation of pressure sores, and act upon them. Prevention is much more dignified, less painful and less time consuming than the complexities of wound management.

There are numerous pressure sore relieving devices and beds available on the market, but these are expensive and not always readily available. Even if you are using these, there is no substitute for a thorough assessment, and prompt action. There are numerous charts available for use to record risk factors, and if these are available you should use them. Whether you use a chart or not, you should consider a number of factors. Is the person experiencing:
– a disease affecting the circulatory system?
– a disease affecting the skin?
– pain which makes it difficult to move around?
– difficulty with weight control (obesity)?
– difficulties maintaining personal hygiene?
– a diet low in the protein and vitamins which help the skin to repair itself?
– excessive use of barrier creams and talcum powder?
– an uncomfortable, hard bed or chair?
– unskilled, outdated manual handling techniques?
– inappropriate positioning?

Make sure that you let the nurse in charge know about any changes in a person's skin condition or ability to get around, so that care plans and charts are always kept up to date.

And finally...

Being able to get around when we want and where we want is something we all take for granted. However, most of us at some time or another have experienced sweatiness and discomfort after a lengthy time sitting down on a hard or vinyl covered hospital chair. If not, you should try it sometime!

If you have ever badly sprained your ankle or broken your leg, you will have also experienced the complete reliance on supportive friends and relatives during your convalescence. You will remember the eternal "clock-watching" and the sheer relief and subsequent embarrassment at the arrival of someone to help you to get on to the toilet.

If this has not happened to you, try and imagine how you would cope for six weeks with your leg in a plaster. Then imagine that you are in a strange place surrounded by people you don't know, with only complete strangers to help you. Finally, think about how it might feel if you also had a poor memory.

Checklist for good practice

1. Daily routines and old habits can contribute to both the conscious and unconscious restraint of people with dementia. Take a look at the everyday practice in your area, to see if this is happening.
2. There are many physical conditions that can affect how much a person is able to get around. It is important to find out about these as soon after they are admitted as possible.

3. You need to get to know someone well in order to explain some of the individual differences which might affect their wish to move around. Always make sure the rest of the team know about these, in order to prevent frustrating misunderstandings.
4. Your verbal and non-verbal communication skills are important. Above all listen and observe. There may be a very good reason why someone is having difficulties.
5. Never force a person to do something which they clearly do not want to do. You may both end up getting hurt. Take the pressure off the situation and come back later, or give someone else a chance to try.
6. Make sure you know where you stand with the law and the manual handling regulations. It is your responsibility to keep up to date.
7. The consequences of an injured back may last for a lifetime. Look after yourself and your colleagues. You may not get a second chance.
8. There are ways of helping people to move around without physically having to lift them. Learn about how the body moves normally and use this knowledge to promote their independence.
9. Remember that the prevention of pressure sores can save everyone a lot of discomfort and indignity. Always assess the potential risk, and make sure everyone knows about it.
10. Imagine how you would cope if you were unable to get around without assistance, and then consider all the things that might make it feel less stressful. How does your practice compare?

Reference
Health and Safety Executive (1992) *The Manual Handling Operations Regulations 1992. Guidance on Regulations.* HSE Books, London.

CHAPTER 11

Restlessness and "wandering"

Brenda Hooper and Tracy Packer

• Lost and restless – how can we help people feel some sense of belonging in a familiar environment? • Observe, search for a pattern, then assess • Some understandable explanations for restlessness and "wandering" • Helpful ways for you to respond • Control and restraint • Relationships

Have you ever lost your car in a multi-storey car park? I remember an occasion when I did so. With increasing desperation, and fighting a rising sense of panic, I wandered up and down the lines of cars. People passed me, walking briskly and confidently straight to their cars. Only I, it seemed, was lost.

I forced myself to try and think logically, to recall at which end of the car park I had come in, and which arrows I had followed. But my wanderings had made me completely disorientated. I had lost all sense of direction. Suddenly, right in front of me, there it was. Oh the relief! I was back in the land of those who knew where they were and where they were going. I almost fell into the driving seat, shaking with the fright I had had.

How can we help people who have dementia, who feel even more frightened and lost, gain some sense of belonging in a familiar environment? An environment which we can take for granted and which gives us our sense of identity?

Some people who appear to be wandering may be obviously distressed or agitated. Others seem calm in themselves as they pace or potter around the room and are sometimes described as "happy wanderers". However, people who do this can unwittingly cause those around them, whether staff or other residents, to be anything but happy! It can be very frustrating for a busy care worker to have to watch apparently aimless and constant restlessness and to feel unable to do anything about it.

Reactions

The way other, mentally alert residents react may be one of the main challenges carers may face. They may become understandably irritated, impatient or distressed by a person who is always "wandering". It is a particular hazard if someone goes into other residents' rooms and disturbs or removes personal items. Most, if not all, people will find it difficult to distinguish between this apparently purposeless moving of objects and deliberate stealing. Frequent accusations of theft on top of the usual trail of mislaid items can seem just too much for hard pressed staff. It is even worse if the person doing the apparent wandering tries to get into someone else's bed!

This raises the issue of whether it is right to care for people who have dementia who also act in ways that appear anti-social to others, in the same setting as residents who are mentally alert. There are no easy answers in the integration/segregation debate. With a comprehensive assessment, many people who have dementia can and do thrive in an integrated environment; although it is never a straightforward issue. Sometimes other residents also prove much more tolerant and accepting than we might expect.

Observe, search for a pattern, then assess

We have acknowledged then, that people with dementia who wander are frequently seen as a considerable problem by care workers. However, there is a variety of explanations we should consider in order to help us understand why somebody is wandering, and then identify the best way of working with it. The first thing to do is to make a careful observation of the wandering activity.

Wandering may appear aimless, and some is, but in certain cases it may be possible to detect a pattern. Does the wandering happen mainly at night, or at a particular time of day, or does it seem to be triggered by some particular event? Beware of too quickly dismissing behaviour as being totally irrational. Perhaps it is possible to imagine how the person is seeing himself or herself at that particular moment in time?

This will lead us on to a consideration of whether there are any discernible reasons for the wandering. Have we any ideas why a person with dementia may wander, or why they wander at the time

they do? To answer these questions it is necessary to have some knowledge of the background and history of the person concerned. The procedures which are eventually put into place will of course also be influenced by the physical characteristics and the location of the home or hospital.

Why do people "wander"?

Losing a sense of one's self

Many people who have dementia stay lost. They never "find the car" but remain disorientated in a world of people who know where they are going. We may have occasional glimpses, like I did in the car park, of what it feels like to be lost, but to live permanently in surroundings that seem strange and unfamiliar is not something most of us have to experience.

People who have dementia are sometimes unable to tell us exactly why they are restless. However, not knowing where you are, what is going on, or what is about to happen – while surrounded by people who clearly do know where they are going and who are moving briskly about their business – can add to the bewilderment, fear and anxiety that a person may feel. In short, psychological restlessness may result in the appearance of physical restlessness.

Restlessness can give us some indication that a person may be feeling as if they have lost the sense of what they *should* be doing and thinking. They may be very aware that things are not the way they should be, and may not be able to put their finger on exactly *what* it is that isn't right. This may offer us some explanation of why people who have dementia can express feelings of disorientation and loss, even when they are in their own home, or in other surroundings that would usually be very familiar to them.

I remember a lady, in the early stages of dementia, standing near the window of her own sitting room and saying in a bewildered voice, "I don't recognise those curtains." She would sometimes also tearfully ask her daughter to take her home. She had never left her home but, spasmodically at first, and finally permanently, she no longer recognised it as her home.

Genuinely lost

It is easy to dismiss the actions of a person who has dementia as those of someone who isn't making any sense or following any logic. One very agile man who was new to a home, tried to get to the communal TV lounge on numerous occasions by walking along the corridor outside his room, opening the fire door, walking across a central courtyard and trying to climb into the lounge through a window. This, of course, caused all kinds of dilemmas, made worse by the fact that on the return journey he always ended up in the wrong bedroom. This distressed both him and his neighbours; and the care workers were at first convinced he was trying to "escape".

He was a very sociable gentleman, who immediately on leaving his private room was able to see the activities in the lounge through the windows overlooking the central courtyard. The corridor to his right appeared long, with identical doors all the way down. For him the quickest way to get to the sociability of the lounge was across the courtyard and if necessary through the lounge window. On the return journey, all of the doors to the private rooms looked the same, so when he thought he was near to his room, he would try the door to every room until he came to the one that looked like his! The solution was to give him a room on a straightforward route to the lounge, and place photographs and other personal items on the door so that he could identify his own room. Unsurprisingly, his "strange wandering behaviour" was curtailed.

It doesn't have to be that complicated. Many people appear to be aimlessly wandering up and down the corridor when in fact they are looking for the toilet, their bedroom, their walking stick, zimmer frame, handbag, or even a place to sit down. One gentleman I knew always got up in the middle of the night to use the toilet. As there was a nightlight by the toilet door he always found it the first time, but was often accused of wandering around the area for a long time afterwards. It became a real issue for the care workers, when he got into the bed belonging to another man who had also popped off to the loo. After a huge fracas on *his* return, it transpired that the first gentleman could not tell the difference between his bed and everybody else's, because all the rooms looked the same. Once a nightlight was put near his bed, the mistaken bed-hopping stopped. People with dementia may not always be able to tell you in words where they are trying to get to, but the more we try to understand their perspective, previous routines, and likes and dislikes, the easier it will be to distinguish a reason.

One final point: try not to fall into the trap of redirecting someone all the way back to a place that is convenient to you. If they haven't found what they are looking for, you will end up doing the same thing every five minutes thereafter with increasing frustration and anxiety for both you and the resident. This will only make an understanding of their actions even more difficult to achieve.

Waiting for something that may or may not happen

Not all residents who wander are necessarily experiencing an acute sense of being geographically "lost". Most of us can remember times when we have been unable to sit still while waiting for an important phone call, or for the postman to bring us a long awaited letter. We have also felt mounting anxiety as the time ticks by and we begin to doubt whether these things will actually take place!

Some people with dementia may take to walking up and down the same stretch of corridor, because they are afraid of missing a visitor they may be expecting. This happens most commonly after a person has been misled by a care worker into believing that his/her relative will "be here soon..." knowing full well that the relative in question is not expected for a couple of days. A person being told untruthfully that they will be having a cup of tea, or something to eat "in a minute...", can also result in them pacing around near the kitchen or dining area.

Some people with dementia may get so excited about a trip out, or worried about missing the taxi/transport, that they get their bags packed and their coat on and pace for hours before the trip is actually due to take place.

In one home, a particular lady was frequently found coming downstairs with her hat and coat on. Staff were frightened that she was about to try and leave the building. What it actually meant was that she had mistaken the day when her daughter was coming to take her out.

Needing to belong

Familiarity with their environment provides reassurance to people who have dementia, even if they have lost the capacity to know where they are, or to remember with whom they live. In a particular home a group of residents had to move to a new building. During the first few weeks one lady wandered a great deal more than she used to in the old building. It was clear that she did not recognise it as her home.

With the passage of time, she wandered less; she had clearly come to feel her surroundings to be more familiar. To help this forward, she had needed lots of reassurance, more staff contact than usual, and her attention directed to her own familiar belongings in her room.

Our sense of belonging in a familiar environment is linked with our own sense of personal identity, so anything that can be done to reinforce that self identification can only help someone to be more at peace in their environment.

A need to escape

Has anyone ever noticed that when care workers have feelings of being rushed, anxious and under pressure, it always seems as if the people with dementia in that setting become equally hassled, anxious and pressurised. No-one is ever sure who was more tense at the outset, but the two groups "mill around" for a while before either something happens to diffuse the tension or a spark is ignited. This spark is usually "fanned" when a person with dementia begins to pace the room expressing clearly that they wish "to go home", or "see my mum". Otherwise they roam around the home trying all the doors (whether private or not), trying to find a way out. The issue is made worse when other residents begin to pick up the increasing tension, and then begin to do the same thing. Pretty soon, the care workers can be overwhelmed by a small "posse" of residents all asking to leave and all wandering around the area.

The next time you come across a similar scene in your area of work, try to "step out" of that situation temporarily and get a feel for the atmosphere at that time:

Is there a high noise level?
Are there lots of people milling about?
Is the phone constantly ringing?
Do the care workers look stressed?
Do the care workers sound stressed?

Do the care workers appear out of control?

If you answer "yes" to just one of these questions, then would it be unreasonable for a person staying there to want to get out to somewhere with some peace and quiet, personal space, no harsh sounds, calm, confident people, and finally, a sense of control and security? Often the use of the words "home" and "mum" at these times is a way of expressing a need to escape to a situation where the comfort, peace and security of "home" or "mum" can protect them from the apparent chaos of the place where they are at this time.

Purposeful or work-like activity

I have witnessed people with dementia on many occasions walking around an area counting the number of doors, tapping the door frames, rearranging files in offices, checking the other residents and moving furniture. This is often related to their previous occupation or routines. Mothers, night watchmen, security guards, housewives, foremen, nurses... The list is endless but these details can have a direct bearing on a person's behaviour, and with a little insight night-time security rounds do not have to be mistaken for inappropriate wandering.

Could this person be an anxious mother, hurrying to pick up her children from school? Does this lady think it is Sunday and she is going to church? One resident always tried to go out at five o'clock in the evening, the time he used to take his dog for a walk.

A patient on an elderly care assessment ward would go into the garden, and then come back and pass urine in the ward. This was because he had lived all his life in a house with an outside lavatory – he had gone out to look for it.

If there is the slightest possibility that someone's wandering activity could be related to their previous work or routines, some creative thinking could incorporate it into a person's daily schedule.

Boredom

Anyone who has waited for a bus that is half an hour overdue can also relate to the repetitive pacing and fidgeting that inevitably seems to take over. But imagine how you might feel if you discovered that there wasn't a bus, that the bus stop was really a nursing home and you could only move around within a 200 metre range at any time. You then discover that there is nothing to do except sit, stand or walk for hours and hours at a time, and the only respite from this are the mealtimes and the dreams you have when you go to sleep.

People with dementia can often be seen walking around and around a unit with no evident purpose. If you can't think of any other reason for this continuous walking, ask yourself this question: *What alternative, fulfilling, activity can this person take part in at this time on this unit?* If you cannot come up with a credible answer, then perhaps the continuous walking taking place is not so unreasonable after all. Maybe then, your team should consider whether providing an alternative would be a worthwhile undertaking (see chapters 1 and 8).

Action

Be calm and validate a person's feelings

How then can we use the information we gain about patterns of wandering and whatever understanding we have gleaned about the residents? Calmness, reassurance, and lots of care worker contact are essential. It may be difficult to treat an apparently "irrational wanderer" as a person with whom one can talk to normally and rationally about the everyday affairs of the home; but to do so may help as nothing else can, to bring this person in touch at that moment with the world about them.

A golden rule is to distract and discuss, not confront. Joining that person for a cup of tea, sitting down for a few minutes to have a chat or to look at some pictures together may have a calming influence, at least for a while. If the person seems determined to go outside, then to go with them for a short stroll around the garden with some everyday conversation may well meet the immediate need. If you think they are feeling lost and out of control, try to reassure the person that you understand a little of what they may be feeling, and attempt to restore calmness, trust and empowerment.

Purposeful occupation to keep boredom at bay

As we have seen, a detailed knowledge of the person's background and previous lifestyle can help. If someone feels the need at five o'clock to go home and prepare the family's tea, then let them help with setting tables, filling milk jugs, etc, for the residents' evening meal.

Being able to go out for regular walks, and being involved with care workers in simple activities for as much of the day as possible, may help enormously. One man who was very disabled by his dementia enjoyed helping the person who does the laundry to fold sheets. In another home, care workers unexpectedly discovered the soothing effect on one of the residents of helping with planting out flowers; they had not previously known that she used to like gardening.

Think about how you are communicating

Remember above all that in talking to people who have dementia, the tone of voice you use may be far more significant than the actual words you choose. If your own irritation or agitation is conveyed to the person who is wandering, this will only make things worse. A calm, friendly, soothing tone will be much more likely to achieve the desired result.

Physical contact, and the way we use it, is as important as speech. The hand on the arm or the arm around the shoulder must convey a gentle desire to lead and to go along with, rather than a forceful pulling against, which will only be counter-productive.

Recognise when you feel vulnerable

Most care workers naturally pride themselves on their patience and understanding. However we are all human, and there will be occasions when we fail to act and speak in as controlled a way as we should. To recognise in ourselves the times when we are at our most vulnerable, and perhaps on occasions to ask another member of staff to help, is nothing to be ashamed of.

We can learn from one another how best to handle particular residents; and sometimes we just have to recognise that, through no fault of our own, a certain person responds better to another care worker than to us. There may simply be something about a care worker that unconsciously reminds the resident of a much loved, or much hated, relative.

Distraction is OK if it is credible

If a resident seems anxious to leave the building, a reasonable suggestion to postpone going outside may sometimes be effective: "There will be a cup of tea soon – why not have that before you go out?" Of course, this does not always work.

One lady started wandering out very soon after she came to live in a certain home. At first the care workers tried straightforwardly to discourage her from going. This merely had the effect of making her angry and resentful. The house was large with several exits and a large garden, and she was clever enough to choose her moment and slip out (often inadequately clothed) by a back way while the care workers were busy elsewhere.

After this had happened a few times, and care workers discovered to their surprise that amazingly she was able to find her way to her daughter's house, sometimes going on a bus, it was decided to pursue a different approach. Care workers tried to be more understanding about her desire to go out (it was partly in response to a family who she felt neglected her). Sometimes they would use the diversionary tactic of a cup of tea, and this often worked. If it failed, they ensured that she had on a warm coat and proper shoes, and that her bus pass was in her handbook. Sometimes she then decided of her own accord that she wouldn't go out after all! Of course her family were also encouraged to visit her more regularly.

Finally, we must not forget the simple fact that some wandering may mean that the resident needs more physical exercise, or is bored!

Control and restraint

Building design
A home with sufficient space for residents to walk around freely indoors without coming to any harm makes management much easier than in a small, confined, cramped building.

There is now an international consensus on good design for dementia care; compensating for the disabilities of dementia with a carefully planned environment. An important principle is "total visual access", which means that wherever they are in a unit, the person can see important areas and join in normal activities. Smaller and non-purpose built homes may of course find it more difficult to provide a suitable layout, but it may be possible to aim towards these principles (see Resources).

Electronic safety aids
There are a number of electronic aids to identification and restraint now on the market. Their use remains controversial. Most are similar to the systems shops use to prevent theft. A small tag is secured somewhere about a resident's person, often as a safety bracelet, and a "pedestal" is placed in any doorway by which they might attempt to leave the building.

When the resident passes the pedestal, their tag completes an electronic loop that activates an alarm system, so that the care workers can bring them back to safety. Those who like the system say it does away with obtrusive and constant surveillance by care workers. Opponents protest that tagging is an infringement of personal dignity, and that its use sets a very dangerous precedent.

Restraining chairs
The use of "geriatric" chairs with clip-on tables, and other physical restraints which are used to prevent people with dementia from getting up and moving freely around the room, can *never* be condoned. They are a denial of the residents' right to freedom and dignity, out of a mistaken sense of responsibility. Special chairs for very disabled people, used with their consent to prevent them falling forward involuntarily, are a different matter.

We must not pretend that these are not difficult and thorny issues.

The use of sedation
The use of sedation is another such question. There are times when a resident's restlessness and wandering is causing them such distress, and is proving so impossible to explain or contain, that some medication may be necessary. This should only be considered when all other avenues have been explored.

Medication must only be given when prescribed by a doctor, and its use and

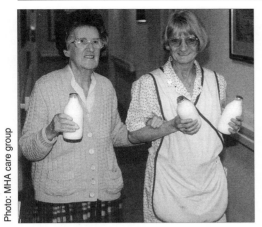

Photo: MHA care group

Going out for regular walks, and being involved in purposeful activities, may help enormously.

effects must be carefully monitored on a daily basis. In particular, minimal use should be made of daytime sedation and it should not be enough to cause drowsiness. It is important to be vigilant when a person with dementia cannot give informed consent to a proposed treatment.

Open doors

Many people doubt whether an open front (and back!) door policy can be justified when caring for vulnerable elderly people who are confused, or who have any degree of dementia. Care workers are understandably anxious about the potential risk to a person with dementia, and are also concerned in case they themselves should be accused by relatives or other people of acting without due care and responsibility. There will be certain rooms inside the building containing hazardous materials etc, which it will be best to keep locked, but it is important that fire exit doors are *always* easy to open.

These are difficult issues. It is important to remember, though, that a person with dementia in care is entitled to the same basic rights as other people. This includes the right to liberty. Elderly mentally frail residents are not normally subject to the compulsory care or treatment provisions of the Mental Health Act. Carers therefore have *no legal right to limit freedom,* and to restrain a resident could be considered an assault or illegal detention. There are certain circumstances where it may be permissible for someone to be physically restrained; for example if it is in self defence, to prevent a breach of the peace, or a crime, or when the consent of the person concerned can be implied or inferred. However, any such action would have to be able to be justified in law.

If a team is sufficiently concerned about a resident's capacity (ability to make a reasonable decision) regarding their own safety, then their manager should approach the doctor responsible for the care of a particular resident and discuss whether there is a need for a mental health assessment to be carried out.

The crux of the matter lies in defining the professional responsibility of care workers for the protection and safety of people who wander, and how this should be interpreted in practice. We must be very careful about assuming that our responsibility to protect a resident from physical harm outweighs the resident's right to freedom to come and go at will.

Whichever approach is adopted will depend partly on the location of the home, and on its nearness to busy roads. However, many homes for people who have dementia do in fact operate an open door policy, and the care workers in one such home commented that the worst consequence any of their residents had suffered was a severe case of sunburn!

What happens when a resident goes missing?

There will inevitably be occasions when a resident does go missing, and every home should have an agreed and written policy for the procedure to be followed. This will vary according to the situation of the home and known patterns of people who are more likely to wander out of the home. Cultivating friendly relationships with neighbours can mean the swift return of a person spotted in the vicinity.

Informing police in advance of people who are likely to be found in the area can be helpful, as can the practice in one home of keeping to hand a description of a "regular" so that only the details of the clothes he was wearing when last seen need be added to the form before handing it to the police. It can be helpful too if people who do wander off carry on their person their name and address; but of course there is no guarantee that a card placed in a wallet or handbag will remain there. Because of this, some form of identity bracelet may be one solution.

Care workers should also carry some form of identification if they are to be involved in following a person with dementia and trying to persuade them to return to the home. This could prevent the embarrassing experience of explaining oneself to a policeman when an apparently lucid resident complains that "this person is following me"!

The importance of communication with residents' relatives must be stressed. It is vital that they are made fully aware of the home's policy about restraint and wandering, and that an anxious son or daughter is helped to understand the reason for the policy.

Relationships

Let us end our consideration on a positive note. However disabled by dementia a person may become and however intractable their wandering may seem, the most constructive approach will always be one that helps to reinforce their own *sense of personal identity*. Wherever possible, have a programme of shared activity. Get residents engaged in simple, everyday things like helping to wash up, clear the tables, go for walks, listen to music, feed the birds. All these things, and more, can help give life within an institutional environment some structure, familiarity and meaning. Establish and strengthen relationships with others, so that people with dementia are seen as individuals by the care workers, who are often the most meaningful and regular contacts.

An open, warm and welcoming atmosphere in all parts of the home or unit, without strict demarcations between staff and resident territory, will provide people who have dementia with the frequent and reassuring contact they so much need.

Checklist for good practice

1. Physical restlessness is linked with mental restlessness, with feeling lost and not belonging.
2. Recent change of surroundings, lack of exercise, boredom, can make wandering worse.
3. Look for patterns, times of day, what triggers it. Try to understand the reasons.
4. Distract, don't confront. Provide simple things to do, with staff.
5. Tone of voice is more important than words used. Be calm and reassuring.
6. Residents have a right to freedom. Physical restraint is difficult to justify. Electronic methods are controversial.
7. Day-time sedation should only be used as a last resort, and should *not* be used if it causes drowsiness.
8. Prepare for what to do when a resident goes missing.
9. An open door approach can work.
10. Be positive. Create a warm friendly atmosphere and good relationships between care workers and residents.

Resource: *Design for Dementia.* Edited by Stephen Judd, Mary Marshall and Peter Phippen. Hawker Publications 1998. (Tel 0171 720 2108).

CHAPTER 12
Personal care and hygiene

Tracy Packer

- *Everyone is different, with their own personal care routine*
- *A good opportunity to observe skills and build up a friendly, trusting relationship* • *Helping with bathing, showering and a bed bath*
- *Hair, skin and mouth care* • *Feet and toes*

Some time ago I heard a nurse tell a story of an elderly gentleman with dementia who refused to have a bath. He had just been admitted to the unit and was so adamant about not having a bath that he would kick and hit out at anyone who tried to get him into it.

Several days went by. He became more and more dishevelled, and the staff caring for him became more and more convinced of his need to have a bath. Every morning they tried, and every morning they were unsuccessful. The gentleman grew more mistrustful of each one of them, and as every attempt failed, the staff became more and more convinced that he was a lazy, dirty, aggressive man. Some even became afraid of him.

Shortly afterwards, a close relative complained to the nurse in charge, about his general appearance. The nurse apologised and explained what was happening. The relative told her this gentleman had only ever bathed once a week on a Sunday evening, because it was the only time he had access to a limited hot water supply. On the other days, he had a thorough strip wash over a basin. Staff took this into consideration, and discovered that he was quite happy to be helped with a daily strip wash. After careful explanations on the following Sunday evening (and every one that followed) he also cheerfully agreed that it would be nice to have a bath.

You will hear, or know of, similar stories as you work in this area of care. They remind us that there are some basic things to consider when helping others to maintain their own personal hygiene needs:

• Everybody is different
Some people like to have a bath or wash every day, others feel that one bath a week is more than enough. Some people may simply dislike baths; others enjoy them but are frightened of being left on their own in the water.

• What works for you may not work for everyone else
It is true that a regular routine helps people with dementia get through

their day with less difficulty. However, well meaning care staff often fall into the trap of sticking rigidly to an established routine. Often this means everybody has a wash or bath when they get up in the morning, and anyone who refuses or does not have one then will go without one until the next day.

It is important (though not always easy!) to find an *individual* routine that works for each person and, if you possibly can, make the organisational routine work around that. Recently on a hospital ward, the night staff bathed one gentleman every night after everyone else had gone to bed. He enjoyed the more restful, less rushed environment and it helped him get a good night sleep. This made everybody happier in the long run.

> **Try to imagine how frightening it must feel, to have your control over something as intimate as washing and dressing taken away from you.**

• **We all like to have some control over our lives**

People with dementia often need more help with simple everyday things. However, there is a subtle but vital difference between taking over and doing everything *to* somebody, and helping out or working *with* somebody to achieve a goal. By working *with* someone, we allow them to have control over what is happening. We can also promote what independence they have, and ultimately the whole experience is much more satisfying and less stressful for all concerned.

Planning ahead

It is surprising how much useful information can be gained about a person's hygiene needs and habits, long before

they enter a bathroom. This information can help identify potential misunderstandings before they could happen. Ask them and their family:

• What was their routine at home **before** they first experienced difficulties?

• Later on, who helped them and how much could they do themself?

• How do they feel about male or female staff assisting them? Often this doesn't matter if it is undertaken with skill and sensitivity, but being sure of this can prevent misunderstandings at a later stage.

• Are there any obvious factors which may affect how good or bad the experience may be for them? For instance:
   – Do they have pain in their joints?
   – Do they have sore feet or toes?
   – Do they suffer from breathlessness?
   – Is their eyesight or hearing impaired at all?
   – Are their gums sore? Do their dentures fit?
   – Do they have sensitive skin/scalp?
   – Do they have any wounds, sores or scars?
   – Are they worried about any disfigurements?
   – What are their continence needs?
   – How good is their balance and co-ordination?

A bit of lateral thinking often helps. One lady I cared for absolutely refused to go anywhere without her handbag. Once we had realised this, we found that bringing it into the bathroom where she could always see it prevented any further problems.

Sometimes people are terrified of water, or have had bad experiences during wash-times. If this is the case, then a great deal of time and patient reassurance may be needed before you can gain their trust. Forcing the issue will make them even more frightened.

The information you need can be gained from other staff who have already been caring for the person, and relatives and friends are often a mine of useful information. But most important is skilled and sensitive questioning of the person themselves and careful listening to what they say and do.

No matter how confused a person may appear to be, often they do try to share things with us, if only we will take time to listen.

Getting ready

Most of the time people are only too happy to wash or bathe, and this can often be the most pleasurable time of the day for them, when they can enjoy your undivided attention.

The principles of washing and bathing are the same wherever they take place, be it in the bed, at the bedside, in a bathroom at a sink, or in a bath or shower.

Take time gathering toiletries, towels, clothes, hair accessories etc, always using the person's own, and encouraging them to help. This is a good time to involve them as much as possible; it helps to give them a feeling of control over their life, and also encourages them to take pride in their appearance.

Try to collect everything that you are likely to need, so that it is all in the wash/bathing area before you start.

Imagine what it would feel like to be sitting in a bath, or half naked by your bedside, when the person you rely on for help keeps disappearing for five minutes at a time to find something...

The area should be warm and draught free, as well as private. This means **no intrusions!** If there is a lock on the door, use it. Actively discourage colleagues from interrupting once you have begun, or barging unannounced through closed curtains and doors.

It always helps to have a small rubbish bag with you so that tissues and disposable cloths can be discarded hygienically. This also helps to avoid the placing of soiled cloths on bedside tables before discarding them, which is an infection risk.

Try to make the whole event as friendly and relaxed as possible. Some people will feel very uneasy about exposing certain parts of their body, particularly the genital area. You need to be discreet and sensitive about this.

Washing and bathing times can be fun, friendly occasions, with a great deal of sociable conversation. Or they can be reduced to mere tasks which need to be efficiently completed, with little or no involvement of the person concerned. Think about the wash times you are involved with. Which category you would put them in?

Remember that washing and bathing:

• provide care staff with the perfect opportunity to assess exactly what a person can do, and where they need guidance or assistance

• offer a good chance of building up a trusting, friendly relationship with the person they are helping. This in turn can help you find out more about the important details of their life and personality

• provide a perfect opportunity for sensory stimulation, with the different textures and smells of the toiletries. A gentle hand or scalp massage could also be given at this time

• enable care staff to make a good all over assessment of skin and joint conditions, and observe for early signs of injury, rashes or soreness

• can influence the mood of a person some considerable time after they are completed. A rushed, sloppy wash may result in a person feeling uncomfortable, disorientated and distressed.

Having a bath or shower

Always ask the person you are helping whether they wish to use the toilet before you begin. Often the sound of running water from the bath triggers off the need to use the toilet. By meeting this need before you begin, you will avoid potential embarrassment and disruption later on.

Once you have everything you need and you are both ready, you can check that the bath is clean and start running the water. (You can always do this beforehand, but take care not to leave it too long as the water will very quickly go cold.) They can then get undressed, or you can assist them in this. Again, try not to leave it too long between helping them to undress and getting in the bath, as the person could become very cold. Be aware that the quality of sound is different in bathrooms, and communicating over the noise of the running water may be more difficult.

Most places now have mixer taps or temperature controls for the water used in bathing. If not, you should always put the cold water in the bath first and then add the hot water. People have been badly burned through getting into a half full bath which only had hot water in it. Always test the temperature of the water with your elbow or forearm (not your hands) before letting the person use it.

The patient may be able to get into the bath with very little assistance, but always use the non-slip mat in the bath if you have one. On many occasions you may have to use a hoist. Do not attempt to lift someone by yourself; always use the equipment provided.

Hoists

Hoists can be very frightening. Be sure to explain what you are going to do **before** you do it, and if possible wrap a large bath towel around the patient's shoulders, while they are in the hoist.

> **Imagine how exposed and frightened you would feel if you were sitting naked in mid air, in an apparently fragile moving chair, not knowing what is happening?**

Keep talking to the person as you move the hoist into position, and tell them when you are beginning to lower the chair. Don't forget to use the brakes at this time. You can still add more hot or cold water at this stage if you want, because the patient will be able to tell you if the temperature is right for them or not by dipping their feet in it. Just before they enter the water you can remove the towel and the chair arms if appropriate, before gently lowering them right down into the bath.

The same principles apply when taking the person out of the bath on the hoist. Let the water out of the bath first and place the large bath towel over their shoulders as soon as you can without getting it wet. This will help to prevent them getting cold on the way back to their wheelchair or chair.

Showering

Not every area has showers available, but they can be extremely useful.

Again, always take care to check the temperature of the water, and if you are using a shower chair with wheels, always use the brakes. Make sure that you do not spray the water directly into the person's face, as this can be distressing and painful.

Always leave the bathroom area clean and tidy, the way you would hope to find it.

Washing by the basin or bedside

If at all possible, hygiene needs should be met away from the bedside. This is not usually a problem if somebody is mobile; if not you can take them in a wheelchair to the washroom area. This will help the person with dementia to remember their daily routine, and the general layout of the care area.

Again, always offer the person a chance to use the toilet before they begin. Check that the sink or bowl you are using is clean before you start, and be sure to change the water when it becomes too dirty or cold. You will also need separate flannels for the face/body, and the sacral/genital areas.

Only ever expose the parts of the body which are currently being washed, and ensure that they are completely dry before putting clean clothes back on. If the skin is at all damp, this can make the whole process much more difficult for the person with dementia, and dressing could become a real dilemma for them.

Giving a bed bath

Bed baths should only be given if someone is too sick to be assisted to sit up and have a wash. Two carers should work together, and if they are well organised, and get everything together before starting, it can be completed in 30-45 minutes. Remember, the more time you take, the more likely it is that the person will enjoy the care and respond favourably next time.

• All of the earlier principles relating to privacy, warmth, communication, preparation and toileting should be applied.

• Both carers should make an effort to include the patient in any conversation, so they are not reduced to the status of an "object" having something done to them.

• Start with the face, and front of the body, keeping areas which are not being washed at that time covered. Change flannels for the groin area and allow the person to wash this area themselves if they are able.

• Change the water, and with the first flannel wash the feet and legs. Then gently roll the person over and wash and dry their back. This is also a good time to change the bottom sheet if necessary.

• Use this opportunity to check that there are no bruises or sore areas over the skin. If you notice any, remember to report this to the person in charge when you have finished. If you are very concerned, cover the person up warmly and gently reassure them, while your colleague finds a senior member of staff to have a look.

• Once you have helped the person to put on clean bed-wear, re-make the bed, check their fingernails, tidy their hair and assist with teeth/denture cleaning. Offer them chance to put on moisturiser or make up if they use it.

Leave the bed area clean and tidy, with all toiletries put away. Clean the washbowl and rinse out flannels before returning them. Ensure the flannels can hang somewhere near to dry. There is nothing more unpleasant than

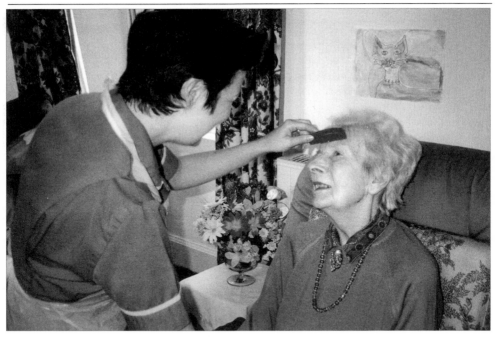

Hair washing and styling can be an enjoyable and relaxing experience.

finding sludgy soap and slimy flannels in the bottom of a toilet bag the following day.

Preventing cross infection

Whichever type of wash you choose to give, be sure to wash your own hands thoroughly between each patient, and change your apron. Aprons not only help to keep you dry, but protect the person from any infections you may be carrying on your clothes or uniform.

Hair care

Hair washing and styling can be an enjoyable and relaxing experience which can help person feel a lot better about themself; or it can be very frightening and traumatic.

Make sure the patient understands exactly what you are going to do before you start. It is best to wash hair over a basin or with a bowl of water on a table. Be sparing with the shampoo and take great care not to pour water into the person's eyes. Make sure the shampoo has been rinsed out thoroughly, then wrap hair and head in a warm towel.

When using a hairdryer, ensure that it is not too hot, and always style hair as requested. If at all possible, get a second mirror so that you can show the finished result from the back. This can often be quite an occasion, so make sure you tell the person how lovely they look, and how much you enjoyed helping them.

Shaving

Most men will have shaved daily throughout their lives. It is important to continue to encourage this where possible, and allow them to do as much as they can for themselves. Whether they choose to use an electric shaver or a razor, be sure never to share these with other people, and always make sure they are clean and dry before putting them away. If your assistance is needed, try to firmly stretch the skin taut, before making a smooth stroke against the direction of the hair growth. Take your time, and be gentle to avoid unnecessary nicks.

Women's facial hair

Some women are prone to superfluous facial hair. This is best removed with a gentle depilatory cream. Always ask permission first, and be sensitive and discreet. This should never be done in public.

Mouth care

Mouth hygiene is just as important as the rest of the body, but often forgotten or neglected. Always provide the means to clean teeth and gums, and offer gentle assistance if necessary. If the patient wears dentures and cannot clean them independently, make sure they get thoroughly cleansed as a part of the daily routine. If someone is very ill and bed bound, a mouth wash and a quick hands and face wash can help to make them feel much fresher.

It is also important to check the mouth and tongue for soreness, bleeding or ulcers. Someone with dementia may not be able to tell you that their mouth is sore, but may hit out in fear of being hurt if you try to clean their teeth or wash their face. Always ensure that dentures actually fit, and that they are clearly labelled and stored in the correct area when not in use.

Nail care

Fingernails should be checked daily and kept neat and tidy at all times. Nails that have not received such care for a long time may be sore and tender or infected. Always ask permission, and explain what you are going to do. If at all in doubt, ask someone more senior to have a look.

Feet and toes

Feet are often neglected by all of us, but there is something immensely pleasurable about soaking our feet in a bowl of warm, pleasant smelling water. This can be done at any time of the day, and allows toenails and hard skin a chance to soften up before trimming. If you are in any doubt about toe nail cutting (for example if the person is diabetic) ask a chiropodist what you can and can't do. As long as you are careful not to cut too close to the skin, and don't try to force tough nailbeds, this should be OK.

Use of toiletries

• Talcum powder can be very pleasant, but it is no substitute for thorough drying. Take care under arms, breasts and in the groin area. Too much powder, especially if the skin is not well dried, will form clumps and cause soreness; and inhaling clouds of talc is not a pleasant experience either.

• Aerosol deodorants can be very cold and quite a shock if the person is not warned before their use. Again take care that the person does not breathe it in.

• Skin care creams are also very soothing, but again they need to be used in small amounts. The more you "slap on" the less effective they are.

It is important that you report any changes (good or bad) in the person's mood, behaviour or abilities, to the person in charge. Remember, information you gain will be useful to others who may care for the same person next time. By passing on what you have learned the information will become part of a written individualised care plan. This will help ensure that maintaining hygiene needs for the person with dementia, will be the pleasant experience it should always be.

And finally...

Always take care of your own appearance and personal hygiene. If you smell of cigarette smoke or have body odour, then the person you assist will not find it a pleasant experience, and may refuse the next time you offer to help them.

Points to remember

1. Everybody is different. We all like to wash at different times of the day, using our own favoured toiletries. Some people are quite content to bathe less often than others.

2. We would all like to stay in control of something as intimate as washing, but some people need more help than others. No matter how dependent on your help a person is, they *never* lose their right to stay in control of this intimate part of their life.

3. The more you know about someone, the more likely it is that you will be working *with* them and not *against* them. If possible spend some time with the person and their family, to find out how they've been coping.

4. Get organised. Always make sure you have everything you will need in one place before you begin. Make sure your colleagues know where you are and ban trivial interruptions.

5. No matter how busy you are, a rushed, sloppy wash may save you time in the short term, but may make the person uncomfortable and irritated; they may even, quite rightly, refuse to cooperate with you next time.

6. Pay attention to details. Mouth and nail care are forgotten or neglected far too often. They are just as important as the main wash.

7. Wash times are a perfect opportunity for sensory stimulation and reminiscence. You are there anyway, so make the most of it!

8. Share any new information or observations with the rest of the team, so that they can benefit when they are caring for the person.

9. First impressions are crucial. The way you help a person to wash and dress makes a direct impression on relatives, visitors and other staff as well. Stand back and take a look. Do the people you have helped look like normal elderly people? If not, why not? What can you do about it?

10. Wash times should be friendly, relaxed and often fun, for both the person with dementia and their carer. If it makes the person feel better, you are allowed to have a good time too!

CHAPTER 13
Promoting continence

Tracy Packer

*• Look at the simple, practical things first • Incontinence of urine
• Indwelling catheters • Pads and continence aids • Incontinence of faeces
Constipation • When accidents happen • A person-centred view*

It is often assumed that as people get older they will automatically experience problems with their bladder and bowels, especially if they have a dementing illness. This is not actually true, but there are a number of issues care staff must consider if they are to help people maintain their continence with greater ease and dignity.

Simple things first

If one of your residents appears to have a continence problem, always eliminate the obvious things first. You will be surprised how apparently simple things can cause great difficulties.

• Are they drinking enough?
In order to keep the kidneys and bladder working and draining well, it is important to drink about two and a half litres of fluid per day. This helps to prevent concentrated urine "stagnating" in the bladder and causing irritation, and it also helps to flush out any infections. (But make sure the person does not have a medical conditions which restricts the amount of fluid they are allowed – check with trained staff first.)

• Are they drinking the right things?
Try to encourage people to drink more water, milk or soft drinks, and less tea or coffee. Cranberry juice is thought to be very good at keeping urine infections at bay. Tea, coffee and cola are better than nothing at all, but contain caffeine which can cause bladder irritation as well as a need to pass urine more often.

Encouraging people with dementia to drink can often be very difficult. Try to be relaxed about it, and leave drinks in strategic places, rather than forcing the issue. Make sure you find out what their favourite drinks are. Those who cannot drink independently are at risk of missing out. Be aware of how much they are getting per day.

• Are they eating the right things?
The right kind of foods in the diet can help to maintain a regular bowel habit. Check that their diet contains plenty of fibre. Fresh fruit and vegetables are rich in natural fibre. You may need to cut up fruit into small pieces on a plate or dish, and again place them about strategically, to encourage some people to eat more. Remember that most fruit

can be blended into delicious milk shake drinks for added variety.

It is also worth remembering that some painkillers and sedatives can increase the risk of constipation. If someone is taking these types of drugs, then you may need to pay even more attention to how much they are drinking and the amount of fibre in their diet.

• How mobile is the person?
Being mobile and active helps food and waste products to to pass through the body. People who are bedbound or unable to move around independently are more at risk of suffering from constipation because waste products do not travel through their system so easily. It is worth remembering this when planning a person's care.

Think about the processes we all have to go through when we use the toilet:

Knowing when you need to go
Does the patient understand when they need to "go"? This might seem obvious, but the process of dementia sometimes muddles up the messages from the brain and bladder so that the person may not recognise the need. Some people may rely on someone else to remind them, or set times when they know they should "go" in order to avoid accidents.

Letting others know
Can the person actually ask someone to help them to the toilet? Someone with dementia may well have difficulty telling you exactly what they want. They may be physically disabled and unable to be able to get out of their chair! They may be in a public place and too embarrassed to ask, or unable to catch the attention of the staff rushing about. Others may not wish to interrupt busy staff, or may be scared of missing something (a visitor, cup of tea or activity) if they go to the toilet.

Finding the toilet in time
Are the toilets clearly signposted? Some people with dementia can no longer make sense of signs with words on them, but recognise symbols. If you couldn't read words, would you be able to find the toilets where you work?

Does the person have the right walking aids and footwear to get there in time. If you are promoting independence, it might be more reassuring and less humiliating to wheel somebody to the toilet and encourage them to walk back, rather than risk an accident.

Do they have to clamber around an obstacle course? The route there, the entrance and the toilet area should be free of excess furniture, rubbish bags etc. The journey may be difficult enough for some people without making it worse. Make sure that those who suffer painful joints or feet, are offered painkillers and well fitting shoes, to help make walking less traumatic for them.

Is the toilet area clean, tidy and warm? Some people will turn around and try and find another toilet, rather than sit on a soiled seat in a smelly room on an unflushed toilet pan. Well, would you use it yourself?

Removing clothing
Clothing can cause all kinds of problems. For example:

• Braces are wonderful when men only want to urinate, because they don't have to try and hold their trousers up as well. However, fumbling with the extra buttons to remove their trousers before opening their bowels, can prove disastrous.

• Velcro on trouser flies and skirt zips, can be a useful alternative for those who cannot co-ordinate their fingers or who are fed up with fumbling around.

• Impossible knots on pyjama cord or complicated belt fastenings, can cause immense frustration and unnecessary accidents.

• Wide skirts and dresses can be more easily tucked into the back of waistbands or lifted up, than tight fitting ones.

• A bulky continence pad can sometimes get in the way if a person spends time fishing it out before using the toilet. If this happens, think about whether the pad is really necessary at all.

Getting on and off the toilet
• Is the seat too high or low?
• Are there horizontal and vertical grab bars that can take the full weight of a person?
• Will their wheelchair fit in the room so they can transfer safely?
• Does the alarm call work?
• Has the nurse forgotten about them?
• Is the door locked?
• Where's the toilet paper?
• How do they turn the taps on at the basin?
• Where are the paper hand towels?
  These are just some of the things that might affect an individual's ability to use the toilet.

Incontinence of urine

Being unable to control where and when you can pass urine is an extremely distressing experience. If this happens to one of your patients, never assume it is part of the process of

dementia and ignore the issue. Always try to establish what is going wrong, and treat the person to whom it has happened with the highest level of privacy and dignity. Reassure them and offer support over what may have been an extremely embarrassing incident for them.

There are a number of reasons why somebody may suffer incontinence of urine:

Urge incontinence
Sometimes the bladder empties just a tiny amount, far too soon and far too often because it is overactive. There are a number of reasons why this happens, but it is always very frightening. Sometimes a patient will refuse to go very far from a toilet because they are worried about this, and they may even make the problem worse by trying to go every ten or fifteen minutes.

It is important to break the vicious circle and try and distract the person for as long as possible before they next go. This takes time; it requires a lot of patience and a great deal of sensitivity. Eventually they may be able to leave it for much longer periods before needing to go.

There are medications available that try to prevent the bladder from behaving this way, which can sometimes be very effective. Be aware that the possible side effects of these may be dryness and a metallic taste in the mouth.

Stress incontinence
This happens when somebody laughs, coughs or sneezes. A small amount of urine leaks out, because the stomach and pelvic muscles supporting the bladder are too weak. There are exercises which can be taught successfully; a thin pad or panty liner may be all that is needed to protect clothes.

Constipation can make this problem worse because full bowels press straight onto the bladder and weaken the abdominal muscles even more, so always check for this. It is also important to offer the chance of more frequent cleansing of the groin area and fresh pads, to prevent soreness, chafing and discomfort.

Overflow incontinence

Constipation, or an enlarged prostate in men, is a common cause of this. The bladder becomes obstructed so that it cannot empty fully. A large amount of urine is left behind and immediately gives the person a feeling of fullness. If this is not recognised, then the urine left behind will stagnate in the bladder. Here it will cause infections, irritation and pain, which could eventually cause kidney damage. Some people find that by gently pressing their abdomen as the urine flow slows, they can empty the bladder further.

Overflow incontinence is often worse at night, and responsible for some episodes of bedwetting. If you suspect this is the problem, a medical assessment may be needed to consider other options.

Reflex incontinence

Sometimes, in dementing illnesses, the messages from the bladder to the brain simply do not get there, or are not interpreted properly. This will result in the bladder simply emptying with no apparent warning.

Never assume that this is the case until you have eliminated all other possible causes for the problem (including all the factors mentioned earlier in this chapter). Infections because of poor daily fluid consumption, are a common and unnecessary cause of this kind of incontinence.

True reflex incontinence may have to be managed with continence aids. Or preferably, it may be possible to anticipate when a person's bladder will empty (and take them to the loo at that time). A special form is used to fill in the details of the amount of urine and the time it was passed, over a period of about a week. It may be possible to identify the times when the person is more likely to go. If staff take this method seriously and offer to take them to the toilet, or remind them just before each time, it can be a very successful way of managing the problem.

Indwelling catheters

A catheter is a tube passed through the urethra into the bladder to collect the urine that gathers there. The urine passes down the tube into a drainage bag attached at the other end.

Catheters are usually inserted by trained nurses or doctors; you should check with them about how they are cared for.

You do need to know that it is important to keep the genital area very clean, to help prevent sending infections up the tube to the bladder. Always ensure that you thoroughly

> **Catheters are an infection risk and should only be considered if all other avenues have been explored, and the loss of dignity to the patient has become intolerable. Catheters should never be an option chosen solely to make the life of care staff easier.**

clean under the foreskin of uncircumcised men, and ensure that you return it over the penis. If you forget to do this the foreskin will swell, causing extreme discomfort and further complications.

Keep the drainage bag below the

level of the bladder at all times, and never block, clamp or restrict the flow of urine through the drainage tube.

Whether catheterised or not, fresh urine should be straw coloured, clear and should not smell particularly offensive. If you are in doubt, or the patient has an unexplained temperature, inform the senior staff, who may request a urine sample for testing.

Catheter tubes and bags may be a source of great embarrassment to those having to use them. Arrange for bags to be emptied before they become too bulky and uncomfortable, and always keep them discreetly covered. If you are not sure how to tie the straps, always ask. Never leave the bag dangling below trouser legs or skirts, this is completely unnecessary and undignified.

Pads and continence aids

Although pads have their uses, their success very much depends on the thoroughness of the assessment of need, and the skill of the practitioner using them. At their worst, pads are expensive, open to misuse, and uncomfortable. Many patients get more satisfaction from pulling them out and tearing them to shreds, than they ever do with regard to their own toileting needs.

If you need to use pads and continence aids:

• Always make sure you have the correct size and absorbency of pad to meet the need. (Do not be tempted to use greater absorbencies than needed, so that the patient can go for longer without having to change.)

• Monitor the patient's skin closely, and report any redness, soreness or broken skin immediately.

• If you do not understand how different catheters, sheaths and pouches

work, then do not embarrass yourself or the patient unnecessarily. Find out as soon as you can.

• Consult your local continence advisor/nurse, so you can be sure you are using the right product in the correct manner. They will also give you invaluable support and advice on assessment and management of different continence problems.

Incontinence of faeces

Constipation

Faecal incontinence does not occur as often as urinary incontinence, but is distressing and unpleasant for staff as well as the person affected. It is most often caused by constipation, when faeces builds up in the bowel and cannot be passed. This can happen for a number of possible reasons:

• The person is not drinking enough, so the stool is hard and dry. This makes it more painful to use the toilet.

• The person does not have enough fibre in their diet, so there is nothing in the stool to stimulate movement through the body system.

• The person is immobile and has weak abdominal muscles which cannot push the faecal matter down through the bowel.

• The person is scared to use the toilet, or is avoiding it because it might involve loss of privacy and dignity, (everyone can hear and smell the results). Or they are afraid of bothering staff who are obviously busy or unsympathetic.

Faecal impaction

Constipation can often be dealt with by addressing these issues. However, it can

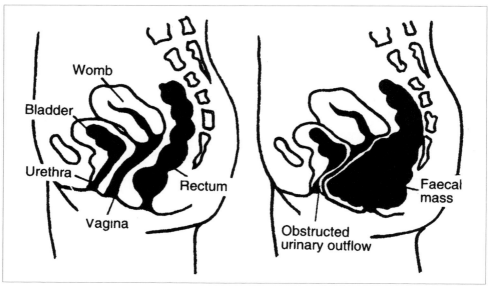

Cross section of female anatomy showing (left) normal bowel and (right) a large mass of impacted faeces.

become so bad that it will result in incontinence of foul smelling, watery, lumpy faeces.

It is important to remember this. Often, incontinence like this is mistaken for diarrhoea, and the unsuspecting patient is given medication to "bung them up" which of course only makes the problem worse.

Many days can pass before an X-ray is taken or the GP called, and the error is noticed. Meanwhile the patient will have suffered great indignities as well as abdominal cramps and pains, nausea and sometimes vomiting, dehydration and loss of appetite.

The overflow happens because the ever-growing build up of hard faeces irritates the lining of the bowel. The irritation causes large amounts of mucus to be produced, which leaks around the edges of the mass, taking small amounts of faeces with it. All the time this is happening, more faecal matter is building up behind, causing more irritation of the lining. Untreated faecal impaction can result in very serious illness.

Faecal incontinence

Incontinence of faeces which has not occurred due to constipation is quite unusual. However, in the later stages of a dementing illness, (and some neurological and spinal illnesses) a few people suffer this, because the brain is no longer receiving the messages from the bowel.

With individualised planning and a regular routine, it may be possible to "plan" when the bowel will be opened. This can either be done through the use of prescribed medicines and/or suppositories. Or it can be integrated into the daily routine, ie about half an hour after a hot drink and some breakfast the person is offered the toilet. Alternatively, sensitive use of suitable pads may be appropriate, but only if there is continuous reassessment of their usefulness.

Accidents

Mishaps do occur for many of the reasons previously mentioned. If someone has an accident, particularly in a communal area, try to appear calm, friendly and reassuring. If a person is afraid of your response, this will only make the situation worse, and increase the chance of it happening again.

Sometimes you will feel disgusted; this is nothing to be ashamed of, and most staff, if they are honest, will admit to sometimes feeling this way. It is important though, to conceal these feelings as much as possible at least while you are dealing with the episode of incontinence.

This can sometimes be very difficult. If you get the chance, it is good to discuss your feelings with other staff, exploring your reactions to such mishaps and thoughts about the way they should be dealt with.

Skin care

A person's skin can become very red and chafed after repeated episodes of incontinence. Always keep an eye out for signs of this around the groin and sacral area. Urine and faeces can cause further irritation and soreness if left on the skin for very long. Always cleanse the genital areas thoroughly; there are now some excellent cleansing lotions and foams available for frequent use with delicate skin.

Why it happened

Once the person has been assisted in their hygiene needs, reassured and returned to their usual routine, it is important to reflect upon why the accident happened. You may discover how to prevent it happening again. Always share this information with other staff, so it can be included in the care plan.

A person-centred view

People all react differently when something as personal as their continence begins to deteriorate, and people with dementia are no exception.

On several occasions I have witnessed people take off an item of their clothing, a cardigan for example, and use it to wipe up the mess. This is wrongly thought to be a deliberate attempt to make the problem worse, when it is actually the person's way of trying to help. They often realise that their "accident" will cause you bother, and attempt to sort it out themselves. Evidence of this sort of help often turns up long after the event, where soiled clothes have been found in bins or obscure places, or blocking a toilet after a failed flush.

Sometimes you will be given little "parcels" of faeces wrapped up in tissues or paper towels. This might appear disgusting, but looked at from the person's point of view, you can see a reason for it. Without the ability to find a toilet or receptacle to get rid of it, they have discreetly wrapped it up for you to take away for them. If they cannot locate someone they feel at ease with, such parcels may stay in a locker or under a pillow for some time!

Often any receptacle around the area will be used as a urinal. This is not necessarily a bad thing, because it shows that at least the patient still knows when their bladder needs emptying. Bins, water jugs, glasses, cups and plant pots are all likely targets. The problem is much more common after dusk, and each person usually has one favoured receptacle.

You can try to take them all away and re-direct the person to the toilet, but this doesn't work very often. The best course of action is to remove potentially inappropriate receptacles and replace them with a container that is. (Making sure it is removed soon after use, emptied and replaced.)

It is also worth considering whether the need for the toilet can explain some of the behaviours associated with dementing illnesses. Ask yourself whether someone might need the toilet if:

• they are getting irritable and agitated for no apparent reason

• they don't sit still, keep standing up and sitting down or wander about aimlessly

• they keep undoing their buttons or flies, or keep taking their trousers/skirt off

• they keep trying doors, and walking into rooms they should not really be in.

Finally, imagine how you would wish to be treated if you were incontinent with no warning, in a strange room full of people that you didn't know? People with dementia are no different from you or I, they feel the same shame and embarrassment, even if they sometimes cannot express it in the same way.

Points to remember

1. Sometimes we miss the most obvious details in the rush to keep someone continent. Think of the simple things first.
2. What a person has to eat and drink is important. Make sure relatives understand this, as they too can contribute to helping with daily fluid and fibre intake.
3. Discussing someone's toileting habits loudly in a communal area, is humiliating to the person concerned. Don't do it!
4. Blank charts with empty boxes on them lead to misunderstanding and poor continence promotion. Always keep bowel and continence charts up to date.
5. If you had no choice but to use the residents' toilets where you work, how would you feel about it? If they aren't good enough for staff, they aren't good enough for **anyone** else.
6. Would you be brave enough to try wearing a night-time incontinence pad for a few hours, and consider how it feels? Perhaps you could pour half a glass of water in it for a realistic effect. Think about this.
7. Never leave catheter bags and tubes dangling in view on the side of tables, chairs, zimmer frames, or under the bottom of skirt or trouser hems. It is not only dangerous but undignified.
8. The next time you have to help clean up someone with diarrhoea, who is not eating much and has been unwell, make sure the team has considered constipation as a possible cause.
9. Did you know that continence advisers can tell you everything you need to know about all brands of catheters, straps, pads, pouches and other aids. Use them.
10. Think about this: You are on your own in a strange coffee bar. Without any warning you are incontinent of urine, and everybody has noticed. You already feel humiliated; what could someone do to make you feel better?

CHAPTER 14

Promoting comfort, sleep and pain control

Cathy Chatten

• The personal touch – individualised care • Physical and psychological causes of discomfort and lack of sleep • How to promote comfort, rest and a good night's sleep • Recognising pain when people don't complain in words, and helping to overcome it • Complementary therapies

We all need to feel accepted as unique, individual human beings. Widely different though we all are, we share a basic psychological need to be understood, accepted for who we are, and encouraged to express ourselves in the way that suits us best.

How then can we as carers meet the psychological and physical needs of people with dementia, when it comes to comfort, rest and sleep? How can we give care which provides for individual tastes and preferences? And how can we ensure that we anticipate and minimise pain or discomfort? The need to get to know each person as an individual, the person-centred approach to care, has been a recurring theme of this book, and is especially important here.

The personal touch

We all need comfort, and we all need to sleep. That much is obvious. But individual preferences and needs vary enormously for our residents, just as they do for us. A lifetime of habit and experiences shapes every resident's needs.

Consider the retired postman, for example, who rose every morning at 5am to begin his round. Maybe he enjoyed a nap in the afternoon, or simply went to bed early to compensate. Dementia may "freeze" those behaviours in time, so that he continues with those habits, even though he now lives in another world. Could we – should we – try to alter this habit of a lifetime in order to fit in with the institutional routine? Not only might it be futile, but it could also create conflict, which in turn could lead to distress and behaviour that is seen as difficult.

Communication difficulties may prevent this gentleman from describing his needs, but the imaginative and perceptive carer will find other ways of discovering which routine would suit him best. Learning all about someone's life history, personality and interests, and planning individualised care, are hallmarks of good practice in dementia care. But we should never underestimate the value of observation and developing a close personal relationship with our residents.

The behaviour patterns are usually there, clearly recognisable, if we are alert to the clues. A baseline sleep chart or day time mood chart will help to reinforce this information. An individualised team approach will give us understanding, and consistency of care. It is infinitely more satisfying for care staff if we can plan care which confirms the individuality of each person in our care, rather than undermines it in the name of routine.

Promoting comfort

Comfort is an important part of health and wellbeing, and it often depends on the ability to adjust successfully to physical, social and psychological change. When planning care we need to think beyond simply avoiding discomfort. We need to think about what life is like in the care environment, how people spend their day, and ways in which we might give practical help and support or maybe provide aids or appliances in specific cases. Helping to preserve our residents' dignity and self-esteem through comfort should always be our aim. We understand now that helping people to lead fulfilling, meaningful lives as opposed to mere existence, is an essential part of our role.

The structure of the average day in a residential setting may owe more to the limitations of the organisation than to the needs of the individuals within it. We know that routines based on physical care can create dependence, purposelessness and disengagement. It is vital that we provide therapeutic activities which meet the psychological needs of our residents, helping them to feel involved in the world around them, and therefore more comfortable and secure.

We all need to feel that we have control over our personal space. Noise, chatter, activity or an over-rigid routine may reinforce feelings of isolation. Personal possessions, a warm, peaceful and familiar environment and a consistent caring approach can help to comfort the troubled mind. Think before you open that window, turn on the radio or even carry out a nursing procedure. We must never forget that for elderly people in long-term care, our working environment is their home. A respectful approach is vital. In everything we do we must constantly keep in mind our residents' right to choose how they live on a day to day basis. We need to work *with* each individual's preferences, never against them.

A good night's sleep

A restful, comfortable day will predispose the individual to a good night's sleep. However, many of the disturbances of sleep pattern associated with ageing become more marked in the presence of dementia. Many people with dementia will:

• Go to bed earlier
• Take a longer time to fall asleep
• Wake more frequently in the night
• Get up earlier
• Take more naps during the day.

Symptoms of anxiety and depression may be particularly noticeable, especially in the earlier stages of the illness. As dementia progresses, reversal of day/night rhythm sometimes develops, with drowsiness during the day and wakefulness from evening onwards. This is sometimes called "sundowning". Lack of daytime stimulation, loss of routine, physical discomfort or unease with one's environment may also contribute to sleeplessness. If you have spent a lifetime sleeping peacefully at night next to your partner, the transition to an unfamiliar room, possibly shared with strangers, will reasonably cause distress.

Many older people rely on night sedation but we know that chemical treatments (drugs) only treat the symptoms, not the cause of the problem. In other words, if the stress of an unfamiliar environment and an uncomfortable bed are the problems, then medication will not make them go away.

We can do a great deal to promote a good night's rest in many instances. We can ensure that preparing for sleep is a natural, pleasant and leisurely ending to the day. Personalised relaxation techniques should be used – as directed by the individual's care plan. A warm bath, for example, and a milky drink may be relaxing for one resident, while the freedom to doze in peace in front of a (relaxing) late night film on television may be therapeutic for another. At all costs, we must avoid imnposing routines which undermine the individuality of our residents.

Warmth, comfort, peace and quiet are basic requirements. Noise should be kept to a minimum, as should sudden alterations in lighting. A bedside commode may help to prevent nocturnal incontinence, provided as part of an individual continence care plan (see chapter 13).

Those at risk of developing pressure sores should be provided with an appropriate pressure relieving mattress, and be regularly but sensitively repositioned during the night to ensure their comfort. Individual choice of bedding may help to make the resident feel more comfortable; some people prefer duvets, others blankets. It should not be beyond the ability of most residential settings to provide for individual taste.

Physical discomfort is a potential source of sleeplessness. It can be avoided very often by careful management of all body functions and physical conditions. A full physical assessment should have been carried out by the nurse in charge and made known to everyone directly providing care. The thorny issue of pain management will be discussed in the next section, as we know it is very relevant when thinking about comfort and sleep.

For people with dementia, a reassuring voice or a friendly touch are of great therapeutic value. The older confused adult may be psychologically vulnerable at night, when sensory deprivation is at its most acute. Night removes many of the clues which help us to make sense of reality. It is our very special duty to be there for our residents, to give emotional support and gently restore wellbeing.

The problem of pain

What is pain? How can we recognise it in others?

Pain involves the interaction of psychological, physiological and social factors. It is a highly subjective experience – it means different things to different people. For the person with dementia, who may be confused and disorientated or have difficulty with communication, this may mean pain is being underestimated and poorly managed. This can create feelings of helplessness and frustration for both resident and carer. An understanding of some of the issues, however, can help to illuminate possible solutions.

It is a commonly held misconception that pain and old age go together. Certainly the older adult is at risk since they are more likely to experience ill health, but pain is by no means inevitable or untreatable. Older people themselves may fail to report their pain, because they are unaware of the benefits that modern health care has to offer. Just as the older adult's attitude toward their pain is affected by their cultural and social background, so might ours be in deciding how best to treat it. Attitudes are often socially learned responses based on our own experiences. How can we really understand what it might be like to feel the pain of arthritis unless we have endured chronic pain ourselves?

Unable to describe or understand their pain, the person with dementia may simply "suffer in silence", or become agitated or restless. Pain can also show itself in sleep disturbance, restricted mobility, apathy, poor concentration, neglect of self care, malnutrition, depression or confusion. These symptoms may mislead us into thinking that the person's mental deterioration is simply gathering pace. What must it be like to be in pain and to be ignored? Treatment of the cause of pain may reduce the likelihood of disturbed behaviour, if we are alert to the clues.

Knowledge of our resident's personality and previous behaviour is the key to recognition of pain, combined with close observation. We should ask our residents and their carers the following questions in order to find out more:

• How does the person describe the pain (if they are able to)?
• When did it start?
• How long does it last?
• Where is it?
• How severe is it?
• What alleviates it?
• Does the pain affect the self care abilities of the person? If so, which ones?
• Does the pain make the person depressed, anxious or angry?

Acute and chronic pain may present themselves differently. Acute pain may produce more obvious signs, which may pass over, whereas chronic pain may produce less obvious signs, but will persist. It has been found that information about pain – what to expect; what might be the causes – can help to increase the sufferer's ability to cope. A person with dementia should be treated no differently. Their inability to respond should not mean they are denied their right to information.

Close personal knowledge can help to anticipate and control some pain. Does the person seem more settled in certain positions? When resting? At certain times of the day? Reducing the situations which might aggravate pain might prevent it becoming more severe. Prompt reporting of any likely signs of pain, even if it is only a "hunch", may help to avoid unnecessary discomfort.

Many of the strategies used to promote comfort and sleep are also useful in this context.

The therapeutic value of touch and a soothing voice should not be underestimated. Reducing sensory disturbances, such as bright light, noise or extremes of temperature can also help. Therapies such as aromatherapy, massage and reflexology are also of value, but they must be used under strictly controlled circumstances. The use of complementary therapies as a method of reducing pain or promoting comfort for the person with dementia will be discussed in the next section.

Selective use of analgesics (painkilling drugs) will help to control some types of acute pain but should always be given for specific conditions, not as a vague "cure all". Some of these drugs will also cause drowsiness, and this will hide symptoms that could lead to correct diagnosis and treatment of an underlying problem. There is also the danger that sedative drugs will obscure the individual's personality. The older mentally impaired adult has a right to sensitive and knowledgeable pain control. They are entitled to individualised assessment and management, which recognises their own unique experience of pain. By using a positive approach, which aims to reduce the physical symptoms and psychological effects of pain, we can make a difference in helping to improve the quality of life for the person with dementia.

Complementary therapies

Complementary therapies use natural, non-invasive techniques, designed for an individual rather than just for a specific medical condition. They may be used alongside orthodox medical treatments or by themselves. They are becoming increasingly popular among health care professionals. In an increasingly technological health culture, complementary therapies seem to provide a gentler approach, creating a closer therapeutic relationship between the therapist and the patient. The emphasis is put on the patient – their tastes, preferences and temperament. A partnership is formed which allows freedom of expression.

Many people who have used compementary therapies speak highly of their beneficial effects. Specific therapies include aromatherapy, massage, therapeutic touch and reflexology. It is beyond the scope of this chapter to describe each of these therapies in detail, but some of the suggested reading at the end of this section may be useful. Although research has yet to demonstrate the "clinical effectiveness" of complementary therapies, many practitioners quote examples of positive benefits for their patients. Research in the field of elderly care recommends a philosophy which considers the whole person, not just their medical symptoms. This may incorporate music, aromas, massage and meditation into an individualised care approach. This can be very empowering both for the carer

Complementary therapies: legal issues

Although the benefits of complementary therapies are clear to many expert practitioners in dementia care, it is difficult to evaluate their effectiveness. Medical research suggests that at best, complementary therapies are not proven to be valuable, and at worst, in the wrong hands they may even be dangerous. Certainly within some healthcare organisations there is a reluctance to adopt complementary therapies as clinically effective practice. So, what are the main issues?

Under the freedom provided by British Common Law, natural medicine has developed further in the United Kingdom than anywhere else in Europe. It is widely used and training standards are high. There are far more restrictions within the European Community as a whole, and with the advent of the common market, they have become part of British legislation.

This could threaten complementary therapies, or it could simply ensure that stricter guidelines are enforced. So far it seems to imply the latter. All complementary therapists are required to have undergone a recognised training programme, in line with other European countries. However, we are still a long way behind our European counterparts in actually standardising and providing this training. In addition, issues such as legal accountability, patient advocacy, health and safety and professional competency must be considered if complementary therapies are to be introduced. Many GPs refer to private therapists, but complementary therapies are practised conservatively in public health care settings, if at all.

or care worker, and for the elderly person. If allowed space, and given the freedom to do so, we can help to soothe the troubled mind of the person with dementia, though positive use of these therapies.

The specific therapeutic uses of complementary therapy for the older adult have been identified as:
• the relief of stress and anxiety
• to provide sensory stimulation
• to calm disturbed behaviour
• as an aid to reminiscence
• as a means of enhancing wellbeing
• as a way of enhancing close relationships between carers and residents
• as an adjunct to terminal care.

Specific treatment-based uses have been described as:
• to alleviate skin conditions
• night sedation
• pain relief
• to alleviate depression
• to alleviate minor digestive disorders.

Most of these approaches use aromatherapy or massage, therapeutic touch, reflexology or a combination of two or more. Essential oils can be administered onto the skin or in the bath. Aromatherapy is by far the most popular therapy. Generally most therapists accept that whichever therapy is used, it will help if the patient believes it will.

Just as we should accept that pain is whatever our residents believe that it is, we should accept that "wellbeing" as an outcome of a therapeutic approach is equally valid. If we have a close personal relationship with our residents, then very often instinct will tell us if a particular therapy is likely to enhance their wellbeing. When used as well as conventional treatment, with full management and family support, complementary therapies can help promote comfort, and relieve stress.

A creative approach

In the past, the fact that there was no cure for dementia has tended to overshadow the many positive things that we now know can be done. Our medical colleagues will often defer to us in psychological care issues, such as comfort, rest, sleep, pain control and use of complementary therapies. Our close personal knowledge of our residents will help to determine our caring approach.

We have many therapeutic techniques at our disposal, but our most valuable allies are empathy and imagination. In other words: our ability to recognise the individual and environmental factors that promote physical and psychological wellbeing, and creatively incorporate them into our care.

Checklist for good practice

1. All care should begin with an individualised assessment, which considers those aspects of the person which go beyond the medical diagnosis.
2. Promoting comfort for our residents is about helping them to adjust to the physical, social and psychological changes of old age and dementia. We must never forget that our working environment is their home.
3. We can help our residents to a restful night's sleep if we respect individual preferences, and are alert to the physical signs of discomfort.
4. Knowledge of someone's personality and previous behaviour is the key to recognition of pain, combined with close observation.
5. Complementary therapies, used conservatively and with supervision, can help to enhance wellbeing in some of our residents, and assist us in promoting comfort.

CHAPTER 15

Loss, bereavement and care of the dying

Jim Marr

• The person with dementia suffers a series of losses, and so do their family and friends • All of them will go through the stages of a grieving process • Care of the dying person • Relieving pain • Spiritual care • An appropriate death

One of the greatest challenges in caring for people with dementia is coming to terms with the fact that despite the very best care we can give, their condition will progressively worsen, and they will become more and more dependent until they eventually require terminal care. Even staff with many years of experience can find this difficult and emotionally challenging. Family and friends who have known the individual for many years may have very mixed feelings about the final period of deterioration: for many it will be a painful, distressing time; but they will also have a sense of relief to know that the person they love is finally at rest and their suffering over.

A series of losses

A person with dementia suffers very many losses, sometimes over a long period of time. Perhaps it begins with a loss of memory and the ability to think clearly, then they may lose their ability to look after themself and perform the normal tasks of daily living. Eventually comes a period when they begin to lose their physical health and require more

and more nursing care, such as help with feeding and drinking. Many people describe this experience as like a jigsaw coming apart. Once there was a whole recognisable picture which made sense, but gradually bits are lost. Eventually the image comes apart to reveal only disjointed pieces which are difficult to recognise.

How family and friends feel

Families and friends often begin to mourn the loss of their loved one long before they have died, and they continue to experience many varied and complex emotions during the course of the illness. They may express this loss by saying things like "that's not my mother anymore" or "my mother would never have said or done that". You know from your reading of earlier chapters in this book that the person *is* still there, and that it is helpful to see any strange, anti-social or difficult behaviour as a form of communication. However, this positive approach can sometimes be very difficult for families to understand. You have an important role in balancing their pessimistic outlook, but you need to be sympathetic to their feelings, which are of overwhelming loss. Sometimes care staff who have looked after a person for a long time may have these feelings too, and begin the grieving process before the person actually dies.

The person's grief

People with dementia may seem to be unaware of what is happening to them, but as we listen more closely and carefully to them we are discovering that this is not the case. They do very often have insight into their condition, but have lost the ability to communicate this to us clearly in words. Some people appear to experience short periods of time when they realise they are failing and become distressed; and sometimes then they can communicate their thoughts and feelings clearly.

But often this distress is seen most clearly in their behaviour, rather than what they say. They may cling to others or seek attention, or even display behaviour which is offensive to others and which is completely uncharacteristic. This may increase distress for their family or friends or make them unpopular with others, and may present an increased challenge to staff to know best how to care for them. Other chapters in this book will help you understand and respond to these situations.

The dying process

In the late 1960s Elizabeth Kubler-Ross, an American doctor, described five stages of dying experienced by the individual and those closest to them. The stages are Denial, Anger, Bargaining, Depression and Acceptance.

Each stage is a method of coping, and gives others an indication of how best to understand and support the person. It is helpful if care staff can learn to recognise each stage, as people do not necessarily experience them in a particular order but may move back and forth according to their feelings at any time. The dying person and those closest to them may experience different stages at different times, and care staff have therefore to be very sensitive in their support. A person with dementia may lose the ability to control their emotions, or they may express their feelings in unusual ways, and they may not understand what is happening, which makes it all more complicated. However, for family and carers these stages may be very real and easily identified.

Denial

In this stage the person denies what is happening and requires support until they get used to the idea of death. They may still have a high degree of hope, believing that recovery is possible, and many will "shop around" seeking opinions and advice from others, or alternative methods of treatment. Staff should understand that this is a normal coping mechanism and offer realistic hope and support, but not lie to them.

Anger

This stage is probably the most difficult for care staff, as anger is frequently directed at those closest to the person. Relatives often say things like, "It's not fair" and "Why should this happen to him/her?" Those involved may feel helpless and frustrated and try to avoid personal contact, but it is important to understand that any criticism or abuse is not directed at care staff personally but at the impending death. It is also important to maintain a pleasant, professional attitude without being either too jolly or morose as either of these extremes are likely to be unhelpful.

Bargaining

This stage is linked to hope; it may last only a short time. It involves seeking ways of postponing the death, often "bargaining" for more time or prolonged life until after a certain event, such as a wedding or the birth of a grandchild. Sometimes poeple may make promises in an attempt to bargain with God for more time or recovery. Sometimes death is seen as a final relief for someone who has had a dementing illness, and bargaining may be about a quick and peaceful death with no more suffering. At this stage it may be very helpful for them to talk to a priest or minister of religion.

Depression

As impending death looms closer and those involved realise that bargaining has failed, a period of loss and regret is experienced. It is clear that the person is emotionally upset, and crying should be seen as a healthy sign of relief of distress. During this period, staff should be aware of the spiritual needs and beliefs of the dying person and ensure that they are visited by a religious representative if this is meaningful for them, and/or their family and friends.

Acceptance

This is a period for saying farewell and tying up loose ends. More distant family and friends may visit for the last time, leaving only those closest to be involved. Physical contact is most important at this stage; touching is very therapeutic especially when those involved prefer to sit in silence, and not to talk. Small gestures of stroking and hand holding can bring comfort, and those closest to the person may ask to be more involved in the care process.

Staff should respect their wishes and encourage and help them to spend time with the person, but it is very important to make sure that they are not left isolated and unsupported.

It is important to remember that these stages are part of a person's unconscious coping mechanisms and those involved may experience them at different times and to different degrees. Some stages may last much longer than others and may still be experienced after the death occurs, during the period of bereavement which can last for up to two years. Staff who are close to the person, and have cared for them over a long time, may experience similar feelings.

Being aware of these stages is useful, but care staff must also always bear in mind that the person with dementia may express their emotions in very different ways from those we normally recognise, and that family and friends are likely to experience mixed emotions including relief as well as regret.

Physical care

As time passes, the individual with dementia will become more and more frail and will require more physical care from staff (see chapter 12). How long this time of increasing frailty lasts will vary greatly from one individual to another; it is always difficult to predict. As friends and family members adjust to the losses dementia brings, attempt to cope with their feelings and plan ahead for the future, they will often ask staff how long the person is likely to live. This is, of course, impossible to say, though the person's general health throughout their life, and any other illness they have, will play a part.

For some individuals, death may come unexpectedly as a result of an acute illness such as pneumonia, heart disease or stroke. As with all sudden death, the shock and surprise for those close to the individual may bring a mixture of emotions even though it was always a possibility. At these times, it is also important to remember that staff may be equally surprised and upset, especially if the cause of death was traumatic – maybe the result of an accident.

Most people with dementia experience a long period of deterioration which eventually involves their physical abilities. They become increasingly dependent on care staff to help them with normal living skills such as feeding, washing, dressing and toileting. Often they become more frail physically, due to weight loss and loss of mobility. Communicating with words becomes more difficult and they may appear to withdraw from others, becoming less responsive.

This can be a difficult time for family and friends when they visit. Staff should be aware of the need to encourage other forms of communication, such as touch, and the need to ensure sensory stimulation. This knowledge should be passed on to visitors. Sometimes something as simple as a favourite tasty treat can then be used to make visits more rewarding for all, and family and friends feel they are doing something worthwhile and meaningful.

Pressure sores

As physical deterioration continues, it is important for care staff to be aware of the possible complications which may occur. If someone is very thin and frail, and cannot move about by themselves, they are at risk of developing sores at points of their body which press or rub against their bed or chair. Special mattresses and cushioning should then be used to help prevent these pressure sores developing.

Food and drink

A nutritious diet (see chapter 9) and plenty of fluids will also help to maintain their physical well-being and prevent problems such as constipation and diarrhoea (see chapter 13). Softer foods may eventually be required to overcome chewing and swallowing problems and sometimes food supplement drinks are needed to ensure that the person is well nourished. At this stage, the family might like to be enlisted to help with feeding difficulties; they may feel more useful and involved if they are encouraged to visit at mealtimes.

Pain assessment

The older person with dementia may not be able to tell you clearly in words when they are in pain or discomfort. Often a change in their behaviour is the only way in which pain is communicated and the individual may "act out" their discomfort or distress.

It is important, therefore, that staff are vigilant for signs which may indicate the need for other care to be implemented. Other indicators of pain may include sounds such as moaning, whining or crying out; facial expressions such as grimacing, clenching teeth or lip-biting; body movements such as restlessness, muscle tension or jerking (see also chapter 14).

If medication is prescribed for pain relief this should be given regularly as ordered by the doctor; but careful positioning, massage and the application of hot or cold compresses may give increased comfort and relief. It is important that any suffering is relieved and an individual assessment is carried out regularly so that pain is controlled. Each individual has a unique response to pain and it is therefore not appropriate to generalise or criticise their reactions.

As a care assistant, you are in a key position to observe, monitor and report this kind of discomfort so that trained nursing staff can act accordingly and give the painkillers the doctor prescribes. Pain assessment charts are often used in these circumstances, but they may not be appropriate for individuals with dementia who are unable to express themselves.

Final stages

Towards the final stages of dementia, increasing frailty and poor health will mean the person needs more rest and sleep. Most of the time will be spent sitting quietly in a comfortable chair. Often reclining chairs are helpful to maintain position and posture when the individual is unable to move by themself.

It is important that attention is paid to areas likely to be damaged by pressure, as sores are just as likely to occur in a chair as in bed. The buttock area is obviously going to be most at risk when someone is sitting for long periods of time, but remember too that the arms should be protected from damage caused by leaning or propping up in an armchair.

At this stage, most individuals will still benefit from the stimulation and interaction of spending time with others in the communal lounge, although a quieter area away from the main activity should be chosen if they become distressed by too much noise and bustle. It is very important to set aside time to sit with the individual and hold or stroke their hand, to maintain therapeutic communication and prevent isolation (see chapter 3). This is something which should be discussed with the family so that they may continue to be involved.

Research has shown that individuals who are very ill are still able to hear what is going on around them even though they do not respond. It is important, therefore, that you continue to speak gently and respectfully, always explaining your actions, even though there may appear to be little feedback.

Spiritual care

Nowadays, we live in a very multi-cultural society. It is very important that care staff are aware of and respect the varied beliefs of those in their care. At the end of life, religious and spiritual beliefs become especially important, as they have a major influence on the individual's attitude to dying.

When a person has dementia they will be unable to organise this support for themselves. Staff should therefore discuss these issues with the family so that arrangements can be made for their minister of religion to visit if appropriate. Often staff can become involved in playing favourite music, such as hymns or other cultural themes, as a method of aiding comfort and support.

Some religions have very specific rituals for the time of death. Your care area should have a set of guidelines so that staff can be aware of these in advance (see chapter 2). The family will also be able to offer help and information. Whatever the situation, it is important that care staff do not impose their own beliefs, or criticise or judge the beliefs of others.

Appropriate death

When someone with dementia is dying it is even more important that staff involved in their care aim to ensure an "appropriate" death. By this I mean that it is the kind of experience they would have chosen for themselves if they were able to do so. A review of the person's life story is useful at this stage, and open discussion with friends and family will ensure that the experience is a fitting final episode to their life. The progression of dementia causes so much of the individual's personality and uniqueness to be buried that other people's memories become increasingly important.

Perhaps in the past some discussions had taken place about funeral arrangements, and the family may have ideas about the person's last wishes. Sometimes, however, care staff have good insight into the individual's desires and can offer relevant suggestions. This is especially true where there has been little family contact, or the final arrangements have been left in the hands of solicitors.

If you have become fond of the person you may well wish to attend their funeral. Senior staff should support this, as it helps you to work through your own feelings. Other residents who have had a close relationship with the person should be kept involved and informed about their condition, and encouraged to express their concerns and feelings as appropriate.

In the last days of life, the individual will usually be cared for in bed in their own room with total help being given. It is important that they are not isolated, however, and an open door and soft music may still encourage contact and stimulation. Family and friends should be encouraged to sit with them as much as possible and to share in their care if they wish. Some may like to read aloud to provide company, some may wish to stay overnight – all of these are entirely appropriate.

Physical care is based around comfort and the prevention of further complications such as pressure sores and infection, so basic care such as gentle changes of position, hygiene, rest and fluids are vital.

Last offices

This is the final act of care which is done for the individual. Experienced care staff may request specifically to perform this care for someone they have looked after over a long period of time, but for an inexperienced care assistant it can be upsetting at first. For the individual with dementia, this is the last stage of loss; and it may be a comfort to family, friends and staff to know they are finally at peace.

Checklist for good practice

1. Dementia is a unique experience for everyone and all must therefore be treated individually.
2. The progression of the disease and the losses experienced vary from one person to the next.
3. Death is also a unique experience for everyone and many different emotions and behaviour may be expressed.
4. In both instances, good communication skills are vital. When verbal communication fails, the importance of touch, facial expression and body language become more important.
5. As physical care needs increase, so too do psychological care needs. Issues of respect, privacy, dignity, protection, safety and rights require special consideration.
6. Emotional support for the patient/client/resident, their family, friends and care staff during deterioration and the dying process is vital.

CHAPTER 16

Behaviour that challenges staff

Michael Maltby

• Describe the problem clearly and exactly • Look for reasons and ask about the past • Can the problem be prevented or tolerated? • Behaviour modification as the next option • Violet – a case example

The aim of this chapter is to offer some general guidance on coping with disturbed and disruptive behaviour. Unfortunately there are rarely any "quick-fix" solutions to behavioural problems. Just because one thing worked with Mrs X does not guarantee it will work with Mr Y!

The only practical way to proceed is to take a step back to assess each situation as fully as possible. Different approaches can then be considered and tried. Even if an effective solution is discovered it will need to be reviewed as circumstances change.

This is essentially a problem-solving process which has to be gone through as each problem arises. In this chapter are some ideas to consider as you work through the main steps listed below:
1. Define what the problem is.
2. Look for any possible causes.
3. Decide what action to take.
4. Take action and evaluate progress.

This is a general approach to follow which can be applied to many situations. It is not possible to go into every behaviour or situation in detail. The specific problems posed by aggression, "wandering" and incontinence are dealt with in separate chapters.

Defining the problem

It is useful to distinguish between:
(a) those things which a person used to do for themselves but can no longer do
    and
(b) those things which some "confused" people may start to do, perhaps for the first time.

To most old people it is what they can't do that is the problem. Being unable to follow a conversation, manage your own affairs or even dress yourself properly can be a source of distress and indignity. However, for those of us offering care, the problem often seems to be what the person starts doing for the first time.

For example, the previously compliant person may start to hit out, resisting all practical help. A quiet, well mannered person may shout and scream for no apparent reason. Another person may start interfering with other people's things, perhaps hiding their own possessions and accusing others of theft.

It is important to keep these problems in perspective. In particular, remember that the problem is not the elderly person themself but what they do. It is easy to label people as "difficult" or "anti-social" but this is usually misleading and unhelpful. Very few people, if any, are difficult or anti-social all of the time. However it can seem that way if we label them in those terms and ignore evidence of other, more acceptable, behaviour.

Perhaps the most positive thing to do is to recognise that all so-called difficult or anti-social behaviour is a challenge to us to find the best way of responding and coping. This avoids labelling the person and makes our task clearer: to respond to the challenge without ignoring the other needs of the person.

No list of such "challenging" behaviour can be complete but some common examples are identified below:

• verbal rudeness, demands and accusations
• repetitive questions and actions
• screaming and shouting
• extreme emotional outbursts and over-reactions
• night-time disturbance/restlessness
• agitation and interference
• hiding and hoarding things
• physical aggression
• self-injuring behaviour
• inappropriate toileting
• wandering
• uninhibited sexual behaviour.

In practice every problem is different and so must be assessed individually. One way of going about this assessment is to ask a series of questions about the behaviour. For example:
What exactly happens?
When does it occur and for *how* long?
Where does it occur?
Who is it a problem for?
How is it a problem for them?

When trying to define a problem in detail in this way, it is important to avoid general statements such as: "He is difficult at meal times." What is needed is an exact description of the behaviour

that occurs and its effects on other people. For example:

"Mr Smith always eats his breakfast quickly and then gets up from his table and takes food from Mrs Jones who is blind and eats slowly. Mrs Jones gets cross and screams out but she can't stop Mr Smith. This upsets the staff on duty who can't always keep a close eye on Mr Smith while serving the food. The problem rarely occurs at other meal times or with anyone other than Mrs Jones."

It may be useful to go through the questions together with everyone involved in the person's care to try and build up a complete picture. Sometimes the results can be quite surprising. A problem that at first seemed huge can be reduced to manageable proportions when you look at it more closely. Perhaps other people don't see it as a problem at all, or have found a way of coping with it.

Looking for reasons

After arriving at a clear description of the behaviour, it is worth trying to understand what the reasons for it might be. This is by no means an easy task, and will sometimes be impossible. You don't need to understand the problem completely before you act. However, the understanding you have is likely to influence what you do, and the way you do it, a great deal.

To blame a person for the way they behave achieves very little and often gets in the way of understanding why they act as they do. This does not mean people should be treated as entirely irresponsible, but the reasons for their behaviour need to be considered first. The behaviour may be the only way a need can be expressed, or may reflect something about the situation which is wrong, rather than the person.

Among the factors which can

contribute to challenging behaviour are:
i) changes in mental functioning
ii) physical and sensory difficulties
iii) social and emotional reactions.

Mental changes

Perhaps the most obvious of these is loss of memory. This might be the straightforward reason why someone keeps asking the same question again and again or forgets where they put something.

Some changes are more subtle but can be just as problematic. For example, lack of the ability to comprehend language may cause someone to misinterpret what is said, and act inappropriately. Some people seem to lose the ability to monitor their own behaviour, so they act on impulse without regard to the consequences.

More dramatic still is the effect of unrealistic beliefs or "delusions" which some people may act on. For example, the belief that other people are after their things may cause a person to hide property, or to lash out at anyone who comes too close.

Physical and sensory difficulties

The effects of pain and physical discomfort can often be masked in an elderly person who can no longer communicate clearly. Instead they may come out as agitated or unsettled behaviour or sometimes as shouting and screaming.

Undetected problems of eyesight and hearing can increase confusion and disturbed behaviour, particularly in an unfamiliar environment. In fact the environment itself can contribute to some problems if it is unsafe, confusing or uncomfortable. The person who strips off their clothes may have no sexual motives but simply feel too hot sitting by a powerful radiator!

Social and emotional reactions

Most people have a strong need to relate to other people and this fact considerably influences their behaviour. As adults we expect to do this with a degree of independence and self-respect. The situation of an elderly "confused" person can be seen as both depriving and threatening in this repect. They have often already lost many of the significant people in their lives and may also have lost control of their own affairs. An awareness of this situation and their own failings can stimulate strong emotional reactions. In the early stages extreme emotional outbursts, sometimes called "catastrophic reactions", can occur as people catch a glimpse of what is happening to them.

Later they may tend to withdraw from social demands or become aggressively independent in an attempt to retain some limited control over their lives. It can be frightening to accept your own needs and trust people to meet them. Far safer, maybe, to resist help and blame others for everything that is going wrong, or alternatively to withdraw completely into your own world.

Ask about the past

Light can sometimes be shone on individual situations by finding out more about a person's previous behaviour from friends and relatives. Current behaviour may be an exaggeration of past patterns or an expression of a particular individual's established needs or fears.

A useful practical approach to any specific behavioural problem is to try and establish if there are any triggers which set if off, or anything that follows it which may make it more likely to happen again. This can be done in the form of an A B C analysis of behaviour where:

A = the Activating event or situation;

B = the Behaviour;

C = the Consequences that follow.

Simply keep a note or think through what happens immediately before the behaviour arises, and what happens immediately afterwards. Does the person get a lot of attention for their behaviour (C), or always react to a certain member of staff (A)? If any pattern emerges, this can go a long way to explaining the behaviour and gives a clue as to what could be done either to avoid or minimise it.

Deciding what to do

Broadly speaking there are three different strategies that can be adopted in the face of challenging behaviour:

i) Prevention

ii) Toleration

iii) Modification.

The first of these is obviously the best. If the problem can be prevented from happening, or at least minimised, everyone is better off. It may be that a problem which can't be prevented can be coped with by making a few adjustments to the pattern of care. Only if prevention or toleration fail should emphasis be placed on trying to change or modify the behaviour itself.

Prevention

Much of what can be done to prevent or minimize challenging behaviour is simply standard good practice in the care of elderly people. Listed below are some of the factors which can make the biggest difference to people who display behavioural problems.

• Maintain *normal expectations*. What you expect a person to do influences the way they actually behave. Look for the best from someone and you are more likely to get it.

• Compensate for *mental disabilities*. Good care involves helping people with what they can't do for themselves. With physical problems this is usually obvious but mental disabilities can easily be ignored.

Anything which helps a person's orientation and sense of belonging is likely to help reduce disruptive behaviour. Using names on doors or labels and signs along corridors can help. Other chapters of this book will guide you in other helpful approaches.

• Encourage *independence* and *activity*. It is often easier to do things for a confused person than let them attempt things themselves. It can also seem very hard to engage them in constructive activity. Unfortunately this can result in frustration and a complete lack of purpose for the elderly person which may fuel inappropriate attempts at activity and independence. Try to get them to do small things for themselves and engage in short periods of activity with other people.

• Avoid any form of *provocation*. This may seem very obvious but is all too easy when time is short and patience is wearing thin. Perhaps the single most important thing is to allow time when you approach someone to tune into their state of mind. A calm, unhurried approach which makes a person feel you are trying to understand them, is ideal.

Toleration

Not all behaviour can be tolerated, but in many circumstances it may be possible to accept it, as long as it does not actually cause anybody any harm. Many forms of sexual behaviour fall into this category. Contrary to popular belief most older people retain their capacity for sexual enjoyment. Inappropriate and disinhibited behaviour may pose problems. However, if the individual has some privacy it need not be unduly disruptive.

Noisy behaviour at night can sometimes be put up with by a careful choice of room, or if rooms are shared, by someone who is hard of hearing!

What is not acceptable is to cope with a person's behaviour by physically restraining them in any permanent way. This is an infringement on the person's freedom. Even in an emergency it is usually better to distract someone, rather than try to restrain them with any use of force.

Some behaviours are so difficult that it may have to be agreed for someone to move elsewhere. This should not be seen as a sign of failure. Some places are more suitable than others for tolerating and coping with particular problems.

Modification

Some forms of behaviour can be changed or made more manageable by the use of drugs, particularly tranquillizers. However these drugs often have unwanted side-effects, and many people are unhappy about taking them. It would seem preferable to try other methods first and to maintain these efforts even when medication is also being used.

Before seeing if it is possible to modify a behaviour, it is necessary to carry out an ABC analysis of the behaviour as described earlier. From this analysis, two possibilities may emerge for changing the behaviour:

a) Altering the activating event or situation (A).

If any event or situation seems to trigger the behaviour regularly, efforts can be made to change the triggering circumstances. Alternatively, a problem may only arise in a certain context, or at a certain time of day, and therefore can be anticipated more easily.

In the example given earlier, where Mr Smith took Mrs Jones' food at breakfast, the trigger could be that Mr Smith has an empty plate and is still hungry. Anticipating this, he could be given a larger portion or a second helping, which might avoid his anti-social behaviour towards Mrs Jones.

b) Altering the consequences that follow the behaviour (C).

This is a deceptively simple thing to do but can be very effective if practised consistently. Many behaviours are maintained by what happens in response to them. For example it is not uncommon for someone to obtain quite a lot of attention for their difficult behaviour. This can be quite rewarding for someone who otherwise might get only limited attention from anyone. In other situations a person may be given cigarettes or food to try and stop them behaving badly. In the long term this is likely to have just the opposite effect!

In fact a behaviour might be repeated again and again just because of the rewarding consequences that sometimes follow it. If this is the case, it can pay to minimise any attention given to the behaviour. This will only work if everyone responds in the same way.

An effort should also be made to provide the reward at another time, when the person is behaving in a more appropriate or acceptable way. If you simply ignore a person's behaviour they are likely to behave increasingly badly to get what they want from you. The idea is to provide the attention, or whatever else they want and need, but only when they are behaving acceptably.

A word should be said about trying to use any form of punishment to alter someone's behaviour. Don't. Apart from being unethical, it is a totally ineffective strategy with most confused people. The emphasis should be on rewarding appropriate behaviour wherever possible.

Taking action

It is often easier to have an idea about what could be done about a behavioural problem than to turn this idea into a plan of action. Every member of staff can try things out for themselves, but this is unlikely to be fully effective unless other people are taking a similar approach. The key is to try and involve as many people as possible at each stage of the problem-solving process. This helps to generate a lot of ideas and means you can agree a realistic plan to follow.

You can rarely expect quick results from anything you try to do. In fact behaviour can sometimes seem temporarily worse when established patterns of care are altered. For this reason it is important to give anything you try a fair chance to work before rejecting it. However, at the end of the day the best approach is to experiment. Try things out and learn from your own experience what works best.

Any measure of success depends on what you are trying to achieve. If your aim is to find ways of making a behaviour more tolerable you wouldn't expect it to go away, but you might hope to reduce its

---

Violet Smith had been a popular resident and had been in the home for about two years. Although sometimes a little confused, she used to recall the past in detail and loved talking to people. However, over the last six months her behaviour had gradually become more of a problem.

At first she just seemed to lose interest in the TV and radio. Then she became more difficult to talk to. Finally she began to shout out for no apparent reason, much to the annoyance of other residents. The more the staff did to try to understand what she wanted the more she shouted, until one day in fury another resident hit her.

The staff wondered whether Violet's hearing might be the problem or whether she had deteriorated mentally. They arranged for assessment which confirmed a significant hearing loss. Tests of mental function showed no further deterioration in memory but found that Violet had developed a problem in understanding and using language. As a result Violet was provided with a hearing aid and staff took increased care to help her communicate.

Violet's behaviour improved. She showed a renewed interest in the TV and radio but still shouted out when they were switched off. The staff decided to monitor her behaviour and found that she only shouted when she had nothing to listen to or occupy herself with. She stopped as soon as someone talked to her. In fact some of the staff would even sit with her when she shouted to stop her upsetting other people.

The staff realised that although her poor hearing and lack of understanding was the original cause of her shouting it now continued as a means of getting much needed personal contact and stimulation. As an experiment they agreed to only give her personal attention when she was not shouting but to do this whenever they could. In addition someone had the bright idea of letting her use a personal cassette player to listen to her favourite music without disturbing other residents.

The results pleased everyone including Violet. She gradually stopped shouting as she found it actually prevented people talking to her. In addition, she obtained great pleasure from listening to music in a way that she had never experienced before.

effect on other people. A preventative approach hasn't failed just because some problems still occur. The best you can hope for is to decrease them.

Similarly, behavioural modification shouldn't be assessed only in terms of the elimination of unwanted behaviours. Any increase in more constructive or appropriate activity indicates considerable success.

With more complex problems, it is well worth trying to keep a written record of the problem and any action taken. This need not be elaborate. A few regular notes or a daily chart is usually sufficient. You can learn a lot about a problem in this way and get a much clearer idea about the effects of what you are doing. It is also helpful to set a date in advance when progress can be reviewed. This gives you something to aim for and ensures that new action can be taken if necessary.

Help and support

With some behavioural problems, the point is reached when professional help may be required to assist with the situation. In addition to the GP, specialist services are increasingly available. These can offer medical and psychological advice on the management of challenging behaviour in elderly people.

It is important to recognise the need for support. Few things are so stressful and emotionally exhausting as caring for people with persistent behavioural problems. Nobody has limitless patience. It is natural to feel angry and upset when your efforts to care for someone are often frustrated. It is all too easy to cope with this by treating some people with less consideration than others. Alternatively your own health can suffer as you struggle to maintain high standards.

The only sensible thing to do is to try and recognise your own feelings. If possible have the courage to be open about them with others. You will usually find other people have experienced something similar and can be a source of support. You can't really expect to care for people whose behaviour is difficult unless you take some time to care for yourself. Chapter 21 explains how you can do this.

Points to remember

1. Try to see the behaviour as a challenge, rather than the person as a problem.
2. Define the behaviour with care. Ask: what, when, where, who, how?
3. Consider carefully what the reasons for the behaviour might be. Take note of mental changes, physical difficulties and social or emotional factors.
4. Remember that prevention is better than cure. So maintain normal expectations, compensate for disabilities, encourage independent activity and avoid provocation.
5. Try carrying out an ABC analysis of the behaviour where: A = the Activating event; B = the Behaviour; C = the Consequences that follow.
6. See if it is possible to change any trigger (A) or rewarding consequences (C) that follow the behaviour.
7. Make an effort to reward appropriate behaviour wherever you can, for example with attention.
8. Before taking any action involve as many people as you can, and try to take a consistent approach.
9. Try things out, and learn from experience what works best by monitoring the results.
10. Recognise the difficulty of the task. In particular be aware of your own feelings and the need for support.

CHAPTER 17

Aggressive and inappropriate behaviour

Valerie Good

• What is aggression and inappropriate behaviour? • Individuals react differently • Understand the causes • How your behaviour and attitude can affect difficult situations • Skills to help you • Responding to aggression – keeping safe • Getting and giving support

These days, following the NHS and Community Care Act, the kind of people in long-stay care settings has changed: they are more dependent and often more confused. This change has led to an increase in the number of "difficult to care for" older people in some units. These people may challenge staff skills by being either abusive, aggressive or by showing inappropriate behaviour.

This chapter looks at ways in which you can play a part in minimising the number of incidents in your unit, and ways of coping with any unacceptable behaviour. It ends with advice about what to do after any incident has occurred. (See also chapters 1, 16 and 18.)

What's the problem?

What is aggression and inappropriate behaviour? It is difficult to find a definition of either aggression or inappropriate behaviour that everyone will agree with. What you find tolerable and what distresses you will depend on your past life experience and your current frame of mind. A good example of this is the effect that different swear words have on people:

some find them offensive and others use them as part of their everyday language.

Aggression can range from verbal abuse through threatening behaviour, such as raising a walking stick, to actual attempts to harm you. Inappropriate behaviour will include clients "making a pass at you", and undressing or masturbating in public areas of the home.

Some people will be admitted to your care already labelled by family or community based staff as being "difficult", others will become "hard to care for" during their stay with you. You will also come across residents who are usually placid and predictable who suddenly act "out of character", displaying some sort of unacceptable behaviour. In order to manage difficult situations better you need knowledge, skill and understanding.

Understand the causes

Few people exhibit difficult behaviour without cause, although it's sometimes hard to understand what the reason was. There are three main causes of unacceptable behaviour: being in pain or under stress, being afraid and through misunderstanding.

Understanding inappropriate behaviour

Most "inappropriate behaviour" is sexual in nature, and in some people is caused by the older person not fully understanding the situation. This would apply to those older people with dementia who start getting undressed in "public" appearing unaware of the other people present. It is also common in dementia for the damage done to the brain to cause *disinhibition* – the spinster may start using sexually explicit language to the embarrassment of her family, or the elderly widower may make a pass at all the women on the staff.

Understand how your behaviour and attitude can affect difficult situations

The way care staff act and relate to residents can directly affect the number and type of aggressive incidents that occur.

Standing too close to people, or towering over them when they are seated, can be intimidating to people whether or not they are confused. It is always better to give people enough personal space and to try always to talk to them at their own level. If they are in a chair or bed, that may mean sitting or crouching down beside them so that your face is level to or below theirs.

Miss Sangster is a 90 year old spinster who has come to your establishment for a fortnight to give her niece a welcome break. On the first evening one of the youngest members of staff, a man of 19, is asked to assist Miss Sangster to bed. They walk arm in arm along the corridor to her room and open the door. Minutes later screams can be heard coming from the room. The shaken member of staff runs out of the room saying "I was only undoing her cardigan buttons"...

Picture Mrs Jones, sitting in an armchair, suffering with chronic arthritis. She has lost most of her language skills and can no longer ask for pain relieving tablets or tell care staff how dreadful the pain is. It's lunchtime and a new member of staff approaches, holds Mrs Jones' arm firmly and pulls her to her feet. Mrs Jones lashes out...

It is late evening. Mr Darby, a recently admitted resident, is trying very hard to find his way to his bedroom unaided. He is a proud and independent man who hates to ask for help. He takes a wrong turn and ends up in the darkened staff room. A member of staff finds him later, sitting in the dark, sobbing. The care assistant says jokingly, "Have you lost your way again Mr Darby?" Mr Darby swears...

Most of us will have experienced angry feelings when someone speaks to us in a dismissive or patronising way. People with dementia are no different. They may take more notice of the tone of your voice than what you actually say; you may be saying something helpful but sounding exasperated and cross, for example. Your body language will also indicate how you feel, and there is evidence that people with dementia who appear to have severe language problems are still aware of body language. Some examples of "unhelpful" body language are talking with your hands on your hips, "wagging" a finger and having your arms crossed.

You need to develop an awareness of the body language you use in different situations. It may help to ask a colleague or friend to watch you and give you some feedback; or a group of care staff may be able to arrange to video each other. Your aim is to find a way of **looking** calm and interested, in control but not threatening.

Ideally your body language, the tone of

your voice and the content of your conversation should all be giving the same message. Your behaviour needs to be respectful, to give residents a sense of their own worth and indicate that you have time for them and **empathy** with them. In other words you need to be able to demonstate to the people you care for, by the way that you work, that you have some idea of what it must be like to be in their situation.

It is important to remember that the way you behave, speak and dress can affect the incidence of inappropriate behaviour. It is not helpful to dress provocatively or to act or talk suggestively.

Residents as individual people

Good care relies on treating each resident as an individual. In order to do this it is necessary for care staff to have a knowledge of each resident and their life and to use this information when compiling the person's care plan. Some people's personalities will seem to have changed as they lose their mental capacities but carers, relatives and friends will be able to provide insights into how the older person dealt with stress and distress in their earlier life.

Consider the difference between the two residents described in the box (right). In trying to provide a high quality of care for both of these residents, you can see that you would need to relate to each of them very differently.

Skilled response

As well as always trying to understand the causes of difficult behaviour, you need a repertoire of skills that will assist you to cope when situations threaten to escalate out of control. Here are a number of ways of responding that you can consider using:
• It may be appropriate to distract the person by diverting their attention to something safer or less distressing (eg by offer-

Mr Adams is a retired bank manager who, according to his wife, ruled his staff with a "rod of iron" and was a stickler for good manners. Mrs Adams and her children had learned not to disagree outright with Mr Adams and had developed sophisticated ways of "getting round him".

Mrs Wright was a delicate child and has been a life long "invalid". She has usually got her own way through emphasising her ill health. She appears timid, easily flustered and never raises her voice. Her husband, who has cared for her for many years, reports that he has found she responds best to gentle teasing and cannot cope with having too many options.

ing a cup of tea, or suggesting looking at the birds feeding in the garden).
• On some occasions it is more appropriate to acknowledge the feelings that lie behind the behaviour ("I know you feel frightened, it must all seem very strange to you..."). Remember that your tone of voice and body language must fit with what you are saying.
• It may be helpful to change course – for example, stop trying to assist someone to get undressed, and let them go to bed fully clothed; or accept that the person does not want their medication now.
• It may be necessary to look at the care environment. Occasionally aggressive behaviour will be triggered by the very design of the home – for example the use of vertical blinds which may be misinterpreted by someone with dementia as bars on the window. Care staff may need to discuss changes with their managers.

Good practice means that it is nearly always best to consider changes to the environment or changes to *your* behaviour, before planning to try and change residents' behaviour.

Responding to aggression

If someone is being aggressive, you must react calmly, taking care not to make things worse either by what you say or do. You may be frightened and want to run away, you may feel like answering or striking back. Your first responsibility must be to assess the situation and try to prevent things getting worse. This may mean removing the older person to prevent them injuring themselves or others; it may mean leaving the situation yourself; or you may need to summon assistance. It is your responsibility to keep yourself safe. You should never attempt to physically restrain anyone unless you have been taught how to by an appropriately qualified teacher.

Keeping safe

There are some simple ways in which you can work towards creating a safe environment in your establishment:
• Never try to rush people with dementia
• Always explain what you are doing
• Never respond to aggression by shouting back or by using threatening behaviour
• You should always know how to summon help if you find yourself in a difficult situation, and you should respond to requests for help from your colleagues promptly
• However stressful your life outside work, you should try to act calmly.

Care plans

As a member of care staff you need to be clear about your responsibilities in relation to care plans. You need to be aware of the practice in your establishment about reading care plans and recording. Care plans should include facts, not opinion, and you need to take care when recording not to mislead. You and your colleagues will not necessarily have the same understanding of some words. For example if you read in a care plan that "Mr Morris is aggressive", what level of difficulty will you expect?

Written and verbal reports need to be clear so that staff can distinguish between someone who is regularly aggressive and someone who has only hit out once; between someone who lashes out with a walking stick and someone who swears. It is very easy to stereotype a resident as being difficult, and by doing so change the way staff relate to them.

Aggression between residents

There will be times when you witness aggression between residents. Your first priority must be to ensure the safety of both parties. You will probably need assistance, and often the solution will be the removal of one resident from the scene for a time. It is important that this is achieved with as much dignity as possible, without stereotyping one party as a troublemaker.

Sometimes the cause of the problem will be clear and there may be ways that it can be avoided in the future: these need to be recorded in the care plan. A frequent cause of aggression between residents will be where people enter the wrong bedroom or sit in the "wrong" chair, or take property not belonging to them. The former problem may be minimised by changes to the environment such as careful signposting and labelling of bedroom doors within the home. Other problems may arise when residents misidentify each other; staff can help by always using residents' names, subtly correcting misidentifications and taking every opportunity to reintroduce residents to each other.

Getting and giving support

There will be times when, despite all attempts to provide good care, there is an aggressive incident in your establishment.

If you were involved you may feel very upset and distressed. It is important that you are able to talk through the situation with a senior colleague. You may need help to learn from the incident, to see if there is anything you could do differently next time.

Often when caring for people with dementia, their aggression is directed at the situation and should not be taken personally. Therefore it is important that you have someone to talk to about how you feel having to continue to care for the person who was aggressive to you. You also ought to be aware of when colleagues need support; sometimes a colleague will need you to take their place while they take some time out to collect themselves.

Finally

You should look upon every incident or potential incident as a challenge, an opportunity to demonstrate your skills as a carer. You need to adopt a problem solving approach, using the techniques discussed earlier in this book. It is unrealistic to aim to eliminate all difficult behaviour: people with dementia have as much right to lose their temper as you do and people with dementia find living in a community as frustrating at times as anyone else would. Your aim should be to make life in your establishment as meaningful as possible for all residents, and to assist residents to express their views and feelings in a variety of ways.

Providing more appropriate activity, giving residents more control over their lives, and being more focused on residents' wishes and less on tasks, will reduce the incidence of "difficult behaviour".

It is very easy to look upon a shift at work as being made up of a series of jobs to be done: beds to be made, bodies to be washed and dressed, and meals to be served. This way of looking at care tends to mean that residents are looked at as objects that need things doing for them. No person is an object, however severe their dementia; it is much better if you can look on work as an opportunity to assist a number of individuals to live their lives to the full, regardless of their disability. It will be easier to do this in homes where there is a key worker system and care staff have a real opportunity to develop a relationship with the people they care for.

Checklist for good practice

1. Don't assume that all elderly people with dementia are difficult or that all older people are incapable of aggression.
2. Don't stereotype people and be careful of the words you use to describe residents to your colleagues.
3. Remember that your tone of voice and body language are as important as what you say.
4. Try to always look for what caused an aggressive outburst. Difficult behaviour does not happen randomly.
5. Always treat people in your care as adults, and as individuals. Be aware of their life history.
6. Be aware of the need to read and update care plans regularly. Care plans should always include information on how difficult behaviour is best dealt with.
7. Try to make sure that the people in your care are pain free, comfortable and occupied. Boredom or inappropriate activity causes difficult behaviour.
8. Don't take aggression personally. Don't feel a failure if you are upset by what has happened; you are only human. Be supportive to colleagues if they are distressed.
9. Concentrate on people not tasks. Do everything you can to highlight people's remaining abilities and skills.
10. Don't take risks. It is your responsibility to keep yourself safe.

CHAPTER 18

Sexuality and sexual needs

Carole Archibald

• Older people are sexual beings and have sexual needs – but staff can find this hard to accept • A framework for action to help you understand "problem" sexual behaviour, and the underlying needs the person may be expressing

Sexuality is about being human: we are all sexual beings. Sexuality embraces such things as close relationships which may or may not include sexual intercourse, kissing, hugging, how we dress, how we laugh, in effect how we present ourselves to the world.

In our world sexual images abound. Whenever we switch on the television, go to the cinema or walk down the street we cannot help but be aware of them. But the images are of young, beautiful and sexy people. You don't see an old man coming out of a lake wearing skin tight Levis or an older woman advertising shampoo. Old age is not what we associate with sexuality. Older people are often considered "past it".

It can be uncomfortable to think of older people – our mothers, fathers, grandparents – being interested in sex, as sexual beings. Yet studies show significant numbers of older people continue to have an interest in, and remain, sexually active. By all accounts they benefit in many ways from this.

For some people sexual expression continues after they are admitted into long-term care. In effect they remain the same people although the environment, in terms of privacy and acceptance of such behaviour, might have changed.

Increasingly in long-term care settings there is a move towards looking beyond the physical needs of residents to their psychological needs: seeing them as persons and acknowledging the uniqueness of each individual. But staff often have difficulty in extending this enlightened approach, this new culture of care, to include residents' sexual needs. This is especially true if a person has dementia.

Is sex a problem?

The expression of sexual need by residents with dementia is seldom seen as a positive aspect of their life. It tends rather to be seen as a problem, something that staff hope will go away, and it is often dealt with in an unsatisfactory way. Sometimes care staff are too embarrassed to mention incidents to colleagues or to the manager.

If the expression of sexuality is seen as a problem then it might be useful to acknowledge this and use it as a starting point to work through situations involving sexual expression in the workplace. The framework for action (p147) which is discussed in my book *Sexuality and Dementia: A Guide* (Archibald 1994)

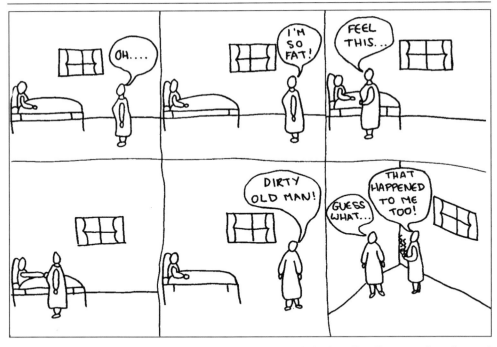

Making a cartoon like this of the situation described below helped staff to discuss and understand what happened, from different points of view, using the framework for action opposite.

offers such an approach. This approach has been found to be useful by staff groups. It gives a clear and structured approach to situations which can, at times, seem out of control, unmanageable and stressful.

The approach is useful because it does not see the problem only in terms of the person with dementia. It allows you and your staff group to look at all the factors which contribute to the situation. The following case study will be used to show how the framework for action might be used and applied to a situation.

Mr B, a man in his late seventies with dementia, has been in residential care for a few months. The reason for his admission was that his wife had died and there was no one to provide the necessary care for him at home. Mr B needs help with dressing and self care.

A young female care worker went into his room one morning to help him get up and dressed. She chatted to him and, amongst other things, told him about the diet she was on, saying how fat she felt. He said, "You don't look too fat to me". Immediately in response she came over to him and placed his hand on her spare tyre round her waist and said "feel that". He did, but his hands did not remain on her waist but sought out and grabbed her breasts.

She was absolutely appalled, went out of his room immediately and reported the incident to the manager. Later at the lunch break she told other care workers, some of whom mentioned similar types of incidents where Mr B had grabbed them. They had never told the manager of these. They felt embarrassed and somehow shamed. They felt a sense of relief in discussing the incidents with each other. Mr B quickly gained a reputation of a dirty old man and was avoided where possible, or only minimum time was spent with him.

FRAMEWORK FOR ACTION

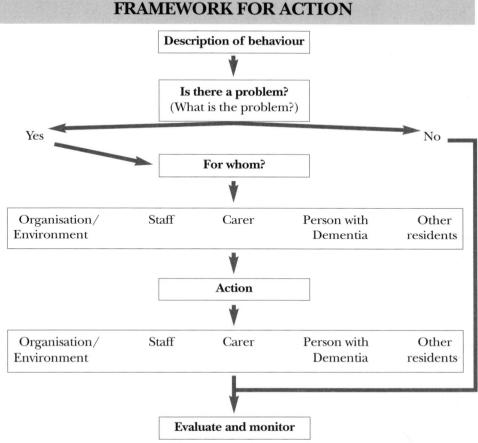

A framework for action – to help staff understand and respond to "problem" sexual behaviour.

Analysing the behaviour

It can be very useful in understanding the situation for staff to cartoon what has happened (see above left). This needs a large piece of paper, ideally a flip chart. Draw lines as for noughts and crosses so that there are six/nine squares. Then one member of staff draws the situation as it happened, using matchstick men. It is useful to draw what was happening before the incident took place, what happened during the incident and what happened afterwards, then to talk through the cartoon applying the framework for action (above).

I have used this with a large number of staff and almost without exception we found it a useful and graphic way of illustrating "the problem", discussing whose problem it is, and helping the staff group look at ways in which they would have changed things if a similar situation occurred again.

Describe the behaviour

There is a need to say simply what the behaviour was, so that staff understand the issues. Here the worker might write "Mr B grabbed the care worker's breasts as she was helping him to get up and ready for breakfast". It can be useful to note down when the situations occurred. This provides a map to help you understand how often and when the incidents happen, and lets you know whether there is a pattern to them.

When you have mapped and recorded this information for about a week, you might think about what the triggers or reasons for the behaviour could be. What was happening at the time, what behaviour resulted and what were the consequences?

Is there a problem?

Once you have looked at the behaviour then you need to ask if it is a problem. If no, there is no further action needed. If the answer is yes, then you need to look at who finds it a problem.

Whose problem is it?

Is it a problem for the organisation?
Has the organisation a policy to ensure not only the rights of residents but to safeguard the welfare of staff? How able do staff feel to talk to managers about issues around sexuality? Are there good lines of communication between staff and management? Is training provided for staff on sexuality and dementia?

Is it a problem for staff?
It would appear from the little information in the case study that staff are clearly upset by events. They report feeling shame and embarrassment and the young care worker was outraged. Is this something staff need to accept? Is there a need to set limits and protect staff, while at the same time helping them to understand the possible reasons for the behaviour, the needs that are being expressed by Mr B?

Are staff contributing to the situation?
Staff not only have difficulty seeing old people as sexual beings, but they also can perceive them as children and react with consternation when old people do not fit this stereotypical picture. Would staff for instance go up to a young male patient/resident and ask them to feel their spare tyre? Would they lean over a younger male in quite the same way they sometimes do with an older resident?

There is another dimension which staff need to think about, and that is the effect of dementia on the person. What's different about dementia? Firstly, people with dementia experience loss of memory. They can forget faces, so that a member of staff carrying out intimate tasks with the person can be misrecognised as their spouse.

The person with dementia may also not recognise themselves as old. Most staff will have experienced residents failing to recognise themselves in recent photographs. If a man perceives himself as young, and a woman is with him carrying out intimate tasks, it isn't too difficult to understand why the resident might respond in a sexual way.

The resident with dementia might not know where they are or what the time is. The front part of their brain might be affected by dementia so that they become disinhibited. They might act in ways they would never have done in the past, approaching people they never would have dreamed of approaching as sexual partners.

While this might not reduce the sense of distaste or make you less embarrassed, it will help in providing possible reasons why the behaviour is occurring. Exploring the reasons why the behaviour occurs also gives the staff group an opportunity to release their feelings and explore their attitudes and reactions to various situations.

Is it a problem for the family carer?

Mr B's wife is dead but he may have relatives who visit. Should the relatives be informed? Should it be an automatic response to inform carers? Are there good reasons why the carer should be involved? These and other questions need to be thought about.

There is little known about how family carers cope with regard to sexuality, particularly partners or spouses. The subject of sexuality is seldom if ever discussed. Where there is a spouse, there may be benefit in the key worker (after first getting to know them and gaining their trust) exploring the nature of the couple's relationship before the onset of dementia, and the difference dementia has made.

From the care worker's point of view, there needs to be an appreciation of the need for privacy and respect for carers who wish to continue their sexual relationship with the resident, if that is what the resident also wishes.

Is it a problem for other residents?

In this case study it does not appear to be a problem for other residents, but in other situations it may be. Their needs have to be considered and questions answered: Is there intimidation by the resident with dementia? Are they distressed by the incidents? Have they complained about unwanted advances?

Is it a problem for the person with dementia - Mr B?

The initial response to this question might be "no". He is getting what he wants. But looking at it further, is he? What he seems to want is some kind of sexual gratification, but what he achieves is little contact. Staff tend to avoid him. So are his needs being met? Clearly they are not.

Developing a plan for action

If our aim is to provide person-centred care, with maintenance of personhood at the core of the action plan, then the care plan should start with the resident.

Mr B

The expression of sexuality is a basic human right – so long as it does not infringe the rights of others. In Mr B's case other people's rights are being infringed, so how should we best address his needs? If Mr B's actions can be interpreted as a means of expressing need, is that need one of touch, need for attention or closeness? If this interpretation is right then he has achieved the very opposite of what he needs!

Is it possible that the more intimate tasks could be carried out by a male worker? If this is not possible, it might help if female staff talked first to Mr B telling him of their husband, boyfriend and/or children, so making sure that he knows who they are and who they are not.

Could the female staff, those who feel able, give Mr B a hand or shoulder massage? To give the right kind of message this would need to be carried out in a sitting area rather than the bedroom. Dancing is another means of giving legitimate touch.

Mr B has only recently lost his wife and if they had a close relationship then he must be sadly missing the physical contact and companionship. Talking about his wife, using photographs and other life story materials, might also be a way of helping him.

The family carer

In this case Mr B's wife is dead. In other situations sensitivity is needed. A skilled person who has built a trusting relationship might explore with the carer their past and present relationships, and on the basis of this information look at ways of helping both the carer and the person with dementia.

This might involve the carer taking the person home for a day, or staff providing a folding bed in the person's room once a week so that the carer can stay overnight. Teaching the carer massage or other activities to encourage closeness needs to be considered if acceptable to both.

The staff

Staff need to feel protected and also need to have some tactics to handle this kind of situation. For example in this case study, if the care worker had treated Mr B like an adult sexual being, she would not have approached him in the familiar way she did. If Mr B did grab out, saying to him firmly "I would rather you didn't do that Mr B" – speaking to him adult to adult, rather than treating him as a child – might be useful way of getting the message across.

Being aware of how staff lean over or bend down near Mr B needs to be considered. Distraction such as singing or reminiscence can be useful, as can giving the person something to hold or fondle (eg a squeezy ball) during intimate tasks.

It is important for staff to examine their own attitudes to sexuality (their own, and that of other groups such as older people). This can be addressed in some measure by training. If staff are to help the person with dementia and their carers they need to feel comfortable with their own sexuality. Sexual expression by residents with dementia can sometimes trigger difficult memories for staff which will affect the way they manage situations. Some sensitive exploration of these issues, by managers or outside organisations, can be helpful.

Other residents

In this case other residents do not seem to be affected. In other situations they might be, so it is important to acknowledge their feelings and address ways of looking at their needs.

The organisation

Some policy to help staff would be useful, as would making sure there are open lines of communication between management and staff so issues can be discussed and brought out into the open.

Resources such as single rooms are needed, so that residents and their carers can have privacy and dignity if they wish to continue their relationship. Resources for staff training are essential so that attitudes and issues can be explored. Resources for activities are also needed so that residents are fulfilled in a meaningful way. The subject of sexuality has for the most part been treated as a taboo subject, so these ideas may be helpful for the organisation to begin to address some of issues.

Monitor and evaluate

When any care plan is made up, it is vital that staff look at whether it has been successful or not. Sometimes there is a need to go back to square one and think again. Sometimes there is a need for some fine tuning. Evaluating whether or not it has been successful can not only be to the advantage of the person with dementia but also it is a learning situation for staff. It can show staff that the initial hard work in going through the framework for action, can pay dividends.

Conclusion

Using the framework for action, instead of immediately reaching for sedatives or removing the person to another place, is hard work. The ideas here do not provide an easy option. They do in fact require more work and a good honest look at ourselves, our own history and attitudes to sexuality, and the way these might affect our responses to the expression of sexuality in the workplace.

But the benefits which come from working through this approach are worth the effort. You, the staff, have a more structured approach which gives direction and provides support. Staff need to talk to each other, to share feelings and views. Residents' needs should be to the fore, and others concerned such as carers and other residents should also have their needs considered. In fact, the needs of all concerned are addressed – a new culture of care in practice.

Further reading/resources

Archibald C (1994) *Sexuality and dementia: a guide*. Dementia Services Development Centre, University of Stirling, Stirling FK9 4LA.
Other training materials on sexuality and dementia, including videos, are also available from the Stirling DSDC. Tel 01786 467740.

Checklist for good practice

1. People remain sexual beings and have sexual needs whatever their age, and whether or not they have dementia. This needs to be acknowledged so that old people, and specifically people with dementia, are seen as adults with accompanying adult needs and desires.
2. Sexual expression by people with dementia can contribute positively to their lives – as long as it is not infringing the rights of others.
3. It is very helpful to explore ways in which people with dementia can express their sexuality, for example through dress, and touch.
4. Education and training is a useful starting point so that you can explore your ideas, attitudes and feelings about sexuality in general, about sexuality in older people, and sexuality in people with dementia.
5. If there is a problem, it is important for all staff to follow a consistent approach, based on a care plan made up by the staff involved.
6. Think about family carers, and other residents. Once you have built up a trusting relationship with them, a private discussion could be helpful.

CHAPTER 19

Relatives and carers

June Andrews and Maria Scurfield

*• All relatives, carers or friends are different • Good reasons
why their involvement is different • They will be anxious, and you can help
• Good and bad ways of communicating • Responding to complaints
• Support groups • Death in the family*

The "relative" of your latest resident may be a husband or wife, son or daughter, nephew or niece, brother or sister, granddaughter or grandson. Or the person who is closest to them might not be a family member at all.

For example, the person who comes and takes most interest might be the man who has lived with your elderly resident for the last twenty years as her lodger. He means more to her than any of her cousins, and you may have much more contact with him than them.

Or it may be that a close friend or partner has lived with the older person for many years, and cared for them with or without help from care agencies.

Whether the person closest to the resident is a relative or not, they may have lived with and cared for them, perhaps for years. For some relatives/carers, care may be satisfying and a source of companionship, for others it can prove to be an exhausting, frustrating and seemingly endless commitment.

Relatives or carers of dependants suffering from dementia are often the hidden victims of the disease. Studies relating to dementia suggest that repetitive behaviours, inappropriate levels of activity, suspicious and destructive behaviours,

sleep disturbances, wandering, incontinence, poor mobility and inability to carry out personal care can cause high levels of stress for both the sufferer and the carer. The decision to admit the sufferer into a continuing care environment is often only a last resort as a result of lack of resources at home. You must not for one moment think that relatives or carers have abandoned the person, or indeed think that they cease to be important because paid health workers have taken on the caring role.

You can see it will not be easy for the carer when the older person is admitted into a home. They are bound to feel a mixture of strong emotions, including:
• relief that the exhausting burden of caring is lifted
• guilt that they could no longer cope
• anxiety that no one else will be able to give the personal care they did, attending to all the little details, likes and dislikes, that are important to the individual
• a sense of loss of purpose or role
• a sense of loneliness, sadness or depression.

If someone is admitted for respite care the same emotions and anxieties are felt. In either case, it is vital that the relative or carer has their views about the person

Relatives and carers:

• **are all different, so their involvement will be different.**

• **may be anxious, and you can help them by anticipating their fears, welcoming questions, finding answers and giving practical information**

• **are often adjusting to a great change, and you are very important in making that possible.**

• **are expert in individualised care if they looked after the resident at home**

• **often get support from each other.**

Remember:

• **the way you tell relatives about the care of elderly residents has a powerful effect on the way they feel**

• **complaints can be a good thing if they are handled sensitively.**

taken into account when the care package is being devised. You need to attend carefully to everything they want to tell you about how the person likes things done. Don't ever assume that you, or other staff, will know best how to care for them just because it is your job.

Individuals

The important thing to remember is that every older person is different, and their relatives are different. Some residents have a close relationship with a family member or friend who cared for them; others have lived alone for many years, and may have no relatives nearby, or even any at all that are still alive.

Think about your own family. There may be some old relatives, for example an elderly aunt, that you send a card to at Christmas, but who lives too far away to visit. On the other hand, your grandma

may live in the same town as you, and be visited each day by a stream of children and adults, so she actually has to get out of the house for a bit of peace and quiet. Then there may be an uncle no one has heard of for years, and you sometimes wonder if he is still alive.

Different relationships

The way the relatives behave towards the home and staff, and the elderly resident, depends on what their relationships have been like in the past.

• "Mum is in a home just three miles from us so we can call round in the car every day, and if the weather is nice, she comes out with us when we go to do the shopping and buys a few bits for herself. When everyone comes to our place for a party, we either fetch her along, or take the party to her, and her friends can see what a big crowd we are and join in the fun. We've almost adopted the women at her place, and they know all of us."

• "I hadn't really spoken to my aunt since I was a child, but as I am a solicitor the family looked to me to make all the arrangements about the home and other financial details. Actually, my brother who is a nurse would have been a better choice. Anyway, they know at the home that they can write to me if there are any problems, but I don't see the point of asking to speak to her. She doesn't know me anyway."

With each of these relatives you can see what the position was before the change of coming into a home. This explains why some relatives have less contact.

Listen for their anxieties

The way people react is very different, but there are a few things you can guess.

If they have experience of what a home is like they will compare you and your surroundings with that. They may have looked at a number of places before choosing yours, so at least you know that you must have some good points.

If they find other things that trouble them, you can do a lot to make them less anxious. They may not ask you directly, but if you listen very carefully to what they say, you may be able to guess their worries.

For example, a son might say, "It's a long way to the dining room from the bedroom". You might think that he was complaining, and think that it is not his problem. You might say, "Yes, and my feet are killing me by the end of the day!"

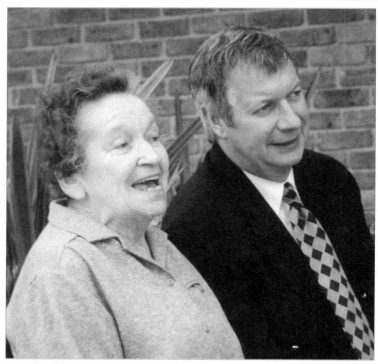

Relationships may well improve following relief from the strain of caring.

But if you listen again you will hear that what he is really saying is, "My dad can't really walk that far in the morning. Will he be all right?" Your answer could be to explain what you do to overcome the problem of the distance, by serving breakfast in bed, or having a buffet breakfast bar where people can get breakfast at any time up till lunch, no matter how slow they are at getting going in the mornings.

You are important

You can also predict that the relatives may be anxious. They may have gone through a great deal of trouble to make this arrangement and they are anxious that nothing should go wrong. When people are anxious they behave in strange ways. Have you ever been to an interview and found yourself laughing nervously at the wrong time and dropping things? Do you remember waiting for ages to see a doctor and then coming out unable to remember what he said, and with a list of unanswered questions in your head?

You might not think if you are working as a care assistant in a residential or nursing home that you make other people nervous, but you should consider the possibility. You are very important to relatives. What you seem to think and feel about their elderly relation can make all the difference between them feeling good or feeling bad about the whole place.

But of course it can work either way. Either the relatives hang on to your every word, and go home and worry about all that you said, or they ignore you and ask to see the person in charge.

If you are always willing to talk, they will eventually discover that you are likely to be able to help or to find out information for them. A word from you about how the resident is doing, or a quote, can make the relative feel better.

• "Janice (she's the little care assistant, who works mornings) says that whenever Dad wakes up he asks for me, and she tells him that I'll be along at the weekend. That keeps me going now. I used to get him up myself, every day, and now he doesn't even recognise me when I sit with him."

Janice is giving the daughter the thanks for all her years of care that she will never hear now from her father himself.

What kind of questions will they ask?
Relatives will often ask the kind of questions that will be answered by this book. Other questions include general information about your residential home that you can answer yourself. Some questions that they ask will seem to have no answer. People might ask about:
• your residential home
• the care of the elderly person
• complaints
• other things that you have to make sure are passed on.

About the home

There may be a leaflet that can be given away that will help the relatives to remember some of the information about your home. If there is not you might be a good person to design it, as the person who does most of the personal care of the resident and therefore has a lot of contact with relatives. You know the kind of questions that can be asked.

Try to fill in this information form from memory, and then ask around to find out the extra information that you need:
NAME OF HOME
FULL POSTAL ADDRESS INCLUDING POST CODE

TELEPHONE NUMBER AND CODE
NAME OF THE PERSON IN CHARGE AND THEIR QUALIFICATIONS
LOCATION: How to get there (maps, and details of public transport might help, and approximate cost of a taxi if necessary).
VISITING: The details of restrictions (if any) or an encouragement to open visiting. Where the visits may take place: in the resident's room, or a private sitting room. Access to the gardens or patio. Whether visitors may take meals by arrangement or make tea.
PERSONAL POSSESSIONS: Can residents bring their own furniture? What security is required? What about insurance, televisions, radios etc. What can be done about labelling, storing and cleaning personal clothing? Can rooms be locked, and is there a lockable cupboard for the resident to keep their private things in?
TIMETABLES: Including details of regular social and recreational activities and outings, times of meals and arrangements to be made for outings, eg packed lunches. Details of local church services.
OTHER: For example who provides any necessary medical cover. Where to get information about fees and pensions and other money matters is also important.

Not least, how to make a complaint.

Ways of telling

When it comes to the care of the elderly person, there are good and bad ways of communicating with relatives:
• "In the morning we get them up and wash them and toilet them. Then we feed them and toilet them again. They get three meals and a cup of tea inbetween and we change them when they're wet. The TV is on for them to watch all the time, and we get them ready for bed after supper. The night staff are supposed to do them twice in the night to see if they are wet or anything. Basically that's it."

• "Hello... How is who?... Wait a minute... Oh, you mean the one who came yesterday in room one?... I've just done that room. She's a bit aggressive, isn't she? Don't worry, we'll take care of that."

Why wouldn't you want to be a resident in that home? Frankly, I don't think you'd even want to work there. What is wrong?

But if you were to visit the home that has been described in this way, it might not be as bad as it sounds. You might find, in the early morning, that some residents are still in bed, some are up and some are quietly getting themselves ready for the day. Of those who need assistance, some are being helped to get washed or to eat and drink, and some are resting quietly.

The atmosphere is calm, but there is a lot of conversation, some laughter, and people listening to each other. People who need help to use the toilet are being helped discreetly. What is the difference?

It is the same place described differently. When relatives ask about the care provided, remember that the way you tell them can influence how much confidence they have in your capacity to care. You can show in your answer that you regard each person as special. When you ring up about your elderly relative late at night it would be better to hear:

• "Hello, Janice Jones speaking. Can I help you?... You want to know about your grandmother who has just come to us. Can you hold on a minute?... Yes, I've just been in to help her settle for the night in her room. It takes a little time to get used to a new place, as I'm sure you know, but you can be certain that we will do everything we can to make her comfortable. Can I give her a message from you...?"

Complaints

The same applies to complaints; there are good and bad ways of handling them. When relatives complain they usually want at least one of three things:
• to get an explanation and an apology
• to get some recompense
• to draw attention to the fact that they are paying attention.

Sometimes the first can be done quite easily:

"This is the third time I have visited and found that my mother does not have her dentures. What kind of place is this?"

It oils the wheels to start by saying that you are sorry that they have been upset in this way, and give an immediate explanation. For example:
– she keeps removing them because they hurt, and she is waiting for a dental appointment for some new ones;
– she keeps leaving them in the toilet when she goes to rinse them after meals, and other residents pick them up (but you have had them marked and you are attempting to keep track of them).

You always have to tell the truth, but a good response includes the reason for the problem, and an indication of what is being done about it. This will often be enough to satisfy the person, but it is wise to let other staff know that the problem exists, especially the person in charge.

The question of recompense rests with the manager of the home, and the owners and insurers. Often people only go on to demand satisfaction if the first stage of apology and explanation is handled badly.

The third item, drawing attention to the fact that they are paying attention, is one which staff often quote to each other.

• "His niece was always in here going on about the food and his clothes and the way we cut his hair. Every little thing and she'd be running to the office. You can tell that she felt guilty about putting him here in the first place".

Some wise person has said that a lot of the anger expressed to staff by relatives is a result of the guilt feelings that they have.

They get over their guilt by letting you know that you are being closely watched.

It is true that when you know that you have done something wrong you may take it out on someone else. It is a short step from slamming the door or shouting at the kids, to picking on a care assistant.

Unfortunately, some staff think guilt is the only explanation for dissatisfaction. Instead of examining what they do in the light of the complaint, they accuse the relative of feeling guilty, and dismiss the complaint without thinking.

Complaints are a good thing. They give you a chance to improve care. Maybe it takes someone's niece to have the courage to say that unless the cook takes a long holiday you'll all die of malnutrition. Relatives' views are valuable and their knowledge may be put to good use.

Complaints also give you the chance to justify the care that you give:

• "I understand that you don't like me calling your mother by her first name, but I have asked her on more than one occasion, and that is what she tells me she prefers."

Give people confidence when you answer their questions. This means:
• Listen very carefully to what they are saying.
• Give an answer if you can.
• Don't be afraid to say you don't know.
• Make sure that they know that you will find someone who can give an answer.
• Make sure that the person in charge knows what kind of thing the relatives are concerned about.

Involvement

Some people want to get very involved in what is happening and some keep well out of the way. How do you feel about this? You might feel that the relative who stays away has dumped the resident, and

SEA VIEW REST HOME FRIENDS GROUP
MEETING 7PM LAST THURSDAY OF THE MONTH
Guest Speaker, Mr Bond from the College of Nursing on the subject of Aromatherapy and Massage
Everyone welcome

Dear Friend,

We are a group of people who are united by having a relative or friend living at Sea View Rest Home. We meet on the last Thursday of every month and have a short talk on subjects related to some of the problems of having a relative or friend in a home. The tea and conversation afterwards usually lead to the next month's topic. We often ask a member of staff to attend.

We have started a car sharing scheme for visiting and are planning a bus trip in the summer. We would be delighted if you would like to come and share both troubles and laughter.
Betty Smith (Chair)

doesn't care. But that may be wrong.

• "I don't go to see mum in the home. Well, the nurses all seem to know what they are doing and I only get in the way. I feel silly just sitting there – she doesn't know me any more. Do you think I'll end up like her?"

As a care assistant you know that older people with dementia appreciate company, even if they do not seem to know who it is. You can tell the relative this, and make sure that they do not feel in the way, as you get on with your jobs.

It is easy to forget, as you do this work every day, that contact with illness or disability (especially dementia) makes many people very anxious. And they do worry about whether a disease runs in the family.

If you realise that they are possibly afraid, you can do the kind of thing that helps in an ordinary way. Let them get involved in activities, make them feel wanted, listen to what they say and make sure that they can get to talk to the person in charge if they need to. Relatives and friends can get involved in many different ways, from helping to serve teas to providing a light entertainment, for example.

• "When our Sarah got married, dad brought the video and slides to show gran at the home. Some of the other ladies showed more interest than gran did, and he goes back once a month now to show his old holiday slides and pictures of us!"

Other relatives seem to show too much interest. Always diving into drawers, turning up at awkward moments and asking questions. But if someone has been taking care of her father at home for years, it can leave a great gap when he goes into a home. She is not feeling guilty, she is feeling lonely, and a bit at a loose end.

You must consider the fact that many relatives or carers will be undergoing intense life changes, especially at the time of admission of the dependant. Relatives and carers are very sensitive to the reactions of staff. A good attitude towards the relative or carer has the potential to reduce their feelings of anxiety. Relatives or carers also seek some form of recognition; therefore by acknowledging their contribution you may increase their satisfaction of caring.

So welcome all the attention! If you are abrupt and avoid questions, they will multiply and come back in greater force. If you answer fully and pay a lot of attention to the person asking, you may find that they are satisfied and turn their attention elsewhere.

Suggest helpful things that the person might do. The really lonely person will love it. The interfering person may back off a little, or even better, find a good channel for their energies.

For most older people, their spouse and their grown children are the most important family members in their lives. If you think about what your family means to you, it is through your family that you maintain ties to the past and future. Families normally provide a sense of personal meaning to life, therefore it is important that they are encouraged to be involved in the life of the person with dementia. Indeed relationships between the relative or carer and the person may improve in terms of closeness because of the relief from strain of caring 24 hours a day.

Your area of work should provide open communication systems for relatives or carers, creating practices that provide a message of welcome to families.

Support groups

When you are going though a difficult period, it often helps to meet with and speak to someone else with the same problem. There are practical as well as emotional problems associated with moving someone into care, and the help and advice that relatives can give each other is invaluable. They may meet by chance during visiting, but sometimes they form a support group. Often a member of staff will get it started in the first place, but then the relatives take it over and run it themselves. They may advertise on a notice board in the home, or by a letter to each new relative (see above).

It is important that support groups are seen as an additional resource. Relatives or carers should not feel that they are an alternative to "one to one" support.

Apart from emotional support, the relatives group can do practical things to help each other and the residents. They are also a great help at the time of a death.

Death in the family

When one of your residents dies you will have a mixture of feelings to deal with. You may feel sorrow and loss, but also happy that you were able to make their last hours comfortable. You will also have to deal with the feelings of the family.

Some people may be distressed because they were not visiting at the time of death. From a practical point of view it can be difficult if the resident is ill for a long time to arrange for them to come at the right moment. The death may be sudden and unexpected, even though the person is old, so the family or friend may have the shock of a telephone call or a message, apparently out of the blue.

It is said that when an old person becomes terminally ill, and perhaps confused or unable to look after themselves,, part of their personality dies. A daughter may say, "That's not my mother talking. She must be feeling awful that we have to do so much for her and she cannot be independent." Carers will often say that it is as if they are already dead. The real person that they know and love has left, and the body left behind is just a shadow of the real person.

So when that person eventually dies, it is a second death for the family. They may say that they feel it is better that the older person is dead; or that they feel relieved because now they can mourn, although the old person died some time before, when they became very ill.

If the relatives come to see the body before the funeral director takes over the arrangements, it helps them if you have shown respect by making the room and the body prepared. You may be asked to help the nurse wash the body and change the sheet, and you may comb and arrange their hair neatly for the last time.

With the room clean and tidy, some flowers and personal things still around, the relatives may wish to sit there alone or with you for a few minutes, just thinking and talking about what has happened and shedding some tears.

Helping with these last duties can be sad, but satisfying. You know you have done your best. Sometimes it is even worse if you come back after some days off and find that an old friend has gone, and there is someone else in the bed.

You can therefore understand how people may feel. They used to visit you regularly and take part in the support group. They don't just lose a relative or close friend, they may lose all the important friendships they had in the home.

This is why many homes make a point of welcoming relatives and friends back after the funeral, for as many visits as they like. The experience of bereavement is something that they can share with the support group. The other residents also may appreciate the chance to talk to them, to express their own condolences, and to continue friendships created through earlier visits.

Checklist for good practice

As a care assistant you have a very important role to play in helping relatives and close friends cope when someone comes to live in the home where you work. The important things include:
1. Remember that everyone is different.
2. The way you describe things is very important.
3. Know what kind of questions will be asked, and how to answer them.
4. Remember how to deal with complaints.
5. Welcome involvement, and try not to judge it.

CHAPTER 20

Ensuring the quality of your care

Lynne Phair

• What is quality? • Ways of measuring quality standards • How you can ensure quality in your own working practice • First impressions are lasting ones • Consider how the older person feels, treat them with respect and offer as much choice as possible • Dementia Care Mapping

Quality has recently become a buzz word in the caring professions. Traditionally, many staff just took it for granted that services gave the best care they could, and therefore never stopped to question the quality of the care they were offering. Now there is a lot of stress on achieving quality standards; but what does this actually mean in practice?

What is quality?

Quality is something that is often intangible – it is unseen as a single item but it is made up of many small parts of a jigsaw. What someone values as quality is in the eye of the beholder, but it should generally be a service which fits the purpose for which it was designed and one that meets the customers needs. In the caring professions, that customer may be the client, the relative or indeed a third party who pays for the care.

Quality should be planned into the delivery of care and established into working practice. Most care environments now have identified methods of ensuring quality and measuring how

quality care is delivered.

Everybody in a team has a role to play in ensuring that older people receive the best care they can have. Ensuring quality should be a commitment of all staff so that a good quality service can ensure:

• a good standard of care for the older person
• a positive and rewarding environment for the staff
• a service that can be offered by the managers with pride and confidence to potential customers.

Quality means different things to different people. In manufacturing, a good quality product is one that meets very clear specifications, which can be measured. The care of older people can never be measured so precisely.

Quality can also mean different things at different times. If you are feeling hungry and want a cheap and quick takeaway, you may feel that the price, the speed and the fact that you can eat it sitting in your car are appropriate to your needs at that time, and so good quality. If, however, you wish to celebrate your anniversary, you may feel that the quality

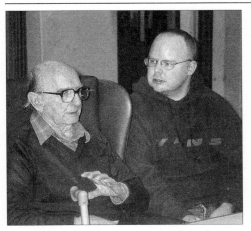

Consideration of how someone feels is the most important aspect of a quality approach to the client that care staff can adopt.

you want is in a restaurant with waitress service and a pleasantly decorated environment. For this you are happy to pay more but still feel it is a quality service. So quality is in the eye of the beholder, and should on the whole be a service which fits the purpose for which it was designed.

What is a quality standard ?

The most important thing to establish is whether the place where you work has got a policy on the type of approach to quality they use. There are a variety of methods, or tools, which measure standards, including British Standard 5750, Total Quality Management, standard setting; and International Standard 9002.

It is not possible, as already highlighted, to state what that quality standard would be for each individual person. There are, however, a number of areas which the staff can address, in their own working practice, that will act as benchmarks for a quality service for older people. As you find out about individual tastes and preferences, and what they enjoy doing, more specific interventions or approaches can be adopted.

First impressions

Think for a moment about the first time you went to a friend's house, or the first time you visited the place where you work. What did you see, feel and think? These first impressions are the most important part of formulating an opinion. What you decided at that time, rightly or wrongly, will stay with you and, if that impression was negative, it will take some time to alter.

When a new resident or their relative visits your unit, their first impression will be what influences them the most. For relatives and the person who may become a resident, the need to feel the warmth of the unit is very important. That warmth is created in the first instance by the first 30 seconds of an encounter. If the care assistant is the first person they meet, that member of staff becomes as important as any of the senior staff or the managers.

Quality practice tips

• First impressions are based on the senses. Staff should think about how others will see them, and what "message" is being given. Staff should show that they have taken care of themselves, that clothes are clean and tidy, their hair is neat in whatever style they choose, their personal hygiene is good – all this shows that staff care about themselves and their work.

• The next positive impression is the facial expression of the staff and their openness in greeting people. It is important to smile and look the person in the eye, and introduce yourself with your name and job title. Always then refer the visitors to the senior member of staff unless you have specifically been given responsibility to look after them.

Quality for the client

For many people who are in the advanced stages of dementia, it may be difficult to discover what they feel is good quality care. There are some ways, however, of trying to ensure that the care offered is at the standard that the person would want.

Consideration of **how someone else feels** is the most important aspect of a quality approach to the client that a care assistant can adopt. The whole of this book has been about valuing each person as an individual: staff should always try to obtain information which helps them to understand the older person and what is important to them. Showing respect in this way will demonstrate that the older person is always central to the care delivered. Part of showing respect is also being polite to the person and showing understanding of their difficulties.

> **Quality practice tips**
> • Show the older person respect by calling them the name they wish to be known by, and don't presume that they will remember your name. Remind them if necessary, gently and politely.
> • Respect the person's property. Personal items should be respected by staff and kept as safely as possible, while always enabling the person to have access to them.
> • Respect the person's privacy by knocking on their bedroom door; don't just enter automatically.
> • Learn about the person as an individual, and help them to do activities and make choices that are important to them.
> • Value the person's property, regardless of how valuable it may appear to staff.

> **Quality practice tips**
> • When the manager informs staff of the policy used in their place of work, it is each member of staff's responsibility to read it and to ask questions about how the unit operates that particular type of quality initiative.
> • If the unit does not have an identified approach to quality, each staff member needs to take personal responsibility for ensuring that a person receives the care they deserve.

It is also important to ensure that the older person is treated with **respect**. When caring for people with dementia, this means always looking to see and respond to the person before the disease. In this way the staff will be able to show respect for and promote the dignity of that person without prejudice. This can be demonstrated in everyday practice.

Remembering that the person may understand what is being said even thought they may not respond, will ensure that staff do not talk across the person. There may be matters that the person would not want discussed in public, and staff should always be mindful that the person may be easily embarrassed even if they can't express it.

However the person responds, staff should always presume that the person's inner feelings will be affected by their (staff's) behaviour, and so should always show respect by not discussing personal matters in a public place. Similarly, the person should always be covered with a sheet while they are being washed or exposed for whatever reason.

It must always be remembered, too, that some people do not want to be cared for by staff of the opposite sex. This could cause problems and upset, and lead to frustration.

For relatives, and the person receiving care, the way the person's property is respected is seen as a measure of the quality of care. Always wash and iron clothes and return them as they should be, and if a person is going home, try to ensure that their property is complete.

The third main way of ensuring quality for the client is to offer **choice**. Everybody in adult life constantly makes choices, whether it is when to get out of bed or whether or not to buy an expensive car. People with dementia will, in most cases, still have an ability to make choices. For some that may be limited, but for others it could be extensive. The choices should be as varied as choice is for the rest of us: choice of food, daily routine, clothing, activity, TV programme, etc. Obviously, in a communal setting, people will have to work together and compromise if there are choices that conflict, but this too is only replicating normal life.

In order to offer real choice to the older person, care staff have to know that person well. This can only be achieved if staff take time to talk with them, and their relatives, and develop a good understanding of what the person likes and enjoys. With this information care staff can assist or guide the person, if help is needed, to enjoy their own individual daily routine Staff should not presume they know best for the older person, without first finding out, or even better, offering a choice.

Quality in the environment

It is not always possible for more junior staff to have control over the environment in which people are being cared for. The environment is, however, an integral part of offering a quality service to older people. Senior staff and managers should be alert and always striving to

Quality practice tip
• Care staff can affect the quality of the environment very positively. Again there is a simple rule to follow: staff themselves should be proud of the environment in which they work.

To achieve this, *everybody* must take responsibility for reporting broken or damaged furniture or fixtures; the home should be kept tidy and dirty crockery always washed promptly. Any spillages should be mopped up immediately and any urinary spillage cleaned and sprayed with a deodoriser, by whoever discovers the problem, not left for the cleaner.

develop an environment that is positive for the residents. They should have the opportunity to plan ahead and budget for large or costly changes.

When someone is admitted to a care home, people are expected to mix and form relationships with others from widely different social backgrounds. The general decor and atmosphere of the unit will also affect people and, if the standard is poor, it will lower their morale and feelings of self worth, and add to their feeling of confusion and disorientation.

Most people need both to spend some time with others, and also have the opportunity to be alone. Older people are no different; a balance of public and private life should be allowed and encouraged.

Measuring quality

There are a number of ways that the amount of quality in a home or ward can be measured. A number of methods of setting the required standard have already been mentioned. These systems may give managers the information they require to ensure that the quality of care

Quality practice tip

Quality is everyone's responsibility. Always listen to what the residents and their families have to say and then think about what they say from their point of view. All complaints should be treated as opportunities to review and improve the care that is given. This does not mean that practice has to change following every complaint, but the issue should be thought about and discussed, either individually with a senior member of staff or, at a team meeting, if the problem is a team one.

in the home continues to reach the standard this client group deserves.

There are a number of other methods that can be useful in developing the way care is given. For example, **Dementia Care Mapping** (DCM) gives a very clear picture of staff's approach to care and the effects on residents' wellbeing. This method of measuring quality identifies many different aspects of care. It maps out what is happening in the home, what is not happening in the home, how the older people receive or respond to the care staff and how the care staff communicate with the older people. DCM highlights the good practice and good communication skills used by staff; it also clearly identifies what areas can be developed through training and education, or changes in routine.

For is more information on DCM, contact Bradford Dementia Group (see *Useful Addresses*).

Some units have meetings at which the older people can make suggestions or comment on issues in the home. Older people with dementia will often not be able to participate; however, some may give clues when they talk to you about things that are concerning them. Always listen to what the person is saying. The words may not be the most important part of the communication. The way the person says the words, and how they look, perhaps anxious or sad, will give clues to what the person is trying to say. Gaining the views of a person with dementia may take time, and snippets of conversation or their actions may need to be collected over a period of time in order to build up a picture of what is being communicated.

Many organisations have official complaints procedures. These are sometimes feared by all staff as the concern is that staff will be chastised if a fault is found. Complaints can and should be used constructively as a springboard for discussion, thoughts and changes, if the complaint is substantiated.

However the quality of care is measured, it is important that the team caring for people with dementia use the information available in a positive way. If the information identifies training needs, or changes in routine, or development in the way people with dementia are cared for, it will ensure that the quality of care continues to improve. Measuring the quality of care in a unit will also highlight good practice, and it is most important that this should always be celebrated.

Points to remember

1. Valuing the older person as someone who deserves respect will automatically improve the quality of care.
2. Staff should be proud of the environment in which they work, taking personal responsibility for reporting faulty equipment, or clearing up spillages.
3. Find out what quality measurement tool the unit uses. Ensure it is understood.
4. Think about how relatives and visitors will view you and other staff. Ensure that your appearance is always clean and tidy.

CHAPTER 21

Stress in your life and your work

Michael Wafer

• What is stress and how does it affect us? • Stress in hospital work • Causes of stress • How to recognise and cope with stress in your life and stressful situations at work • The patient's point of view • Special problems for women

There seems to be a general view in our society that life today is more stressful than it was many years ago. But what is stress?

We all know when we experience it, but may have difficulty defining it. The word is derived from "distress", and when used in a day-to-day sense we think of being under pressure, under strain, and lacking energy.

In a medical sense the term means the release of chemicals within the body, providing extra energy for either "fight or flight". In primitive times, if a person felt threatened in his surroundings the body would respond by providing enough extra energy to run away or to fight.

In our day-to-day life we also have threatening experiences. An example might be going to the dentist: our primitive response to the threat is to run away, and our body provides us with the chemicals to do so. Most of us, however, remain sitting in the chair. The chemicals released still have an effect on the body: an example of an illness caused by this process is stomach ulcers. Indeed, it is recognised that many modern diseases are caused in part by stress.

Stress can also be pleasurable and useful. We can feel stressed when watching a horror movie, riding on a roller coaster or watching our team at Wembley. When feeling stressed we sometimes give our best performance through a "burst of adrenalin". This type of beneficial stress is sometimes called *eustress*.

Stress and dementia care

It is generally accepted that working with people with dementia can be stressful. This is partly to do with the nature of the work, such as the close contact with people who may be distressed or difficult to communicate with.

In addition relatives of people with dementia may be anxious and have difficulty coming to terms with their relatives' conditions. Other reasons can be working shifts, low pay, poor working conditions or fear of job loss.

These feelings of stress have very important consequences. They may make people less effective in their work, so the care given to others suffers. Stress at work may also affect people's personal lives and close relationships. It is therefore in everyone's interest that stress is understood, and limited.

What causes stress?

Researchers have tried to identify **events in life** which are particularly stressful. These include, in order of severity:
• Death of partner
• Divorce or separation
• Death of close family member
• Marriage
• Loss of job
• Gain of new family member
• Financial problems
• Change in housing
• Change of job.

If you have experienced one or more of the above within the last twelve months it is likely that you have felt under some degree of stress.

Examples of **work situations** which may make you feel stressed are:
• Dealing with seriously ill patients
• Not feeling valued as a team member
• Being asked to do tasks for which you have not been adequately trained
• Difficult relationships with senior staff
• Sexual harassment
• Witnessing bad practice.

In addition there are many other factors in the workplace which can make us feel stressed. These include difficult staff relations, medical emergencies, and too much noise.

A particular problem for the care assistant is that because of your position in the organisation you may feel relatively powerless, with no control over the things putting you under strain. The truth is, of course, that you do have control over what happens to you at work, and you can influence the people around you and the environment. Some of the ways you can do this will be discussed later.

Recognising stress

If you are suffering from stress, your body will tell you! Some physical symptoms include feeling sick, sweating, going to the toilet more often, irregular periods, constipation, dry mouth, inability to sleep, indigestion, eating more or eating less, headaches, and palpitations.

In addition, you may have alterations in mood. You may cry more easily, feel down and depressed, anxious, inadequate, negative or hysterical. You may not be able to think clearly, lack concentration, be unable to make decisions, feel that your life is totally out of control.

Stress may also be evident in a change of behaviour, such as absenteeism, arriving late for work, increased smoking and drinking, being withdrawn and quiet, inappropriate laughter, being aggressive or clumsy. Sometimes others will recognise you are under stress before you do.

Coping with stress

In trying to cope with stress there are three broad approaches. You can try and live your life so that your body is not exposed to unpleasant and unnecessary stress; or try to identify the cause of stress and eliminate or reduce it; or try and deal with the feelings produced by stress.

Lifestyle
In order to reduce stress you should try and lead a healthy lifestyle. This includes paying attention to your diet – not only should it be "balanced" (including a wide variety of good food) but you should not miss meals. This can be particularly difficult for people working irregular hours. Try to reduce your intake of tea and coffee and drink fluids without caffeine as it is a stimulant and may contribute to your feeling stressed.

It is important to get enough sleep.

Allow for adequate rest times: if you have any influence on work rotas try to avoid working for long periods without days off; similarly try to take holidays at equally spaced intervals.

Exercise is very important. Not only will it make you fitter, it will help you work off stressful feelings and also sleep better.

In addition to a healthy lifestyle it is important to find ways to relax. These are very personal but might include listening to music or going for a walk.

Talk to someone

A very important way of relieving and preventing stress is talking about it. Find a suitable time to confide in someone you trust about the things which are making you feel stressed. Sometimes friends and partners may provide the support you need, but can find it difficult to understand work-related problems. Often work colleagues can be very supportive.

Some employers provide counselling within the occupational health service, or via independent counsellors. In addition you may find voluntary organisations helpful, for example MIND (the National Association for Mental Health), Relate (Marriage Guidance), and the Samaritans, whose local numbers can be found in the Yellow Pages telephone directory.

Find the cause

If you are feeling stressed you should try to identify the cause. You cannot always remove the cause, of course, but in some instances you can. You may be stressed because of high noise levels for example, which you might be able to reduce.

A common cause of stress is difficulty with colleagues; if so, it is important to talk with the person concerned. In the short term it may feel uncomfortable, but it is likely to have long term benefits.

Smoking and drinking

Unfortunately many of us deal with the problems of stress by alleviating the symptoms – increasing our alcohol intake, or smoking more. This may make us feel better for a while, but once the drink has gone the problem will still be there (and may be made worse by a hangover).

Stress in the workplace

Perhaps the single most important factor in reducing stress in the workplace is the development of good relationships between workers; which is not always easy to attain.

An important element of good working relationships is **trust**. The following will destroy trust:

• talking critically behind people's backs
• breaking confidences
• breaking agreements
• trying to manipulate people
• being inconsistent
• reporting to a senior person without discussion with the person concerned first.

Trust can be developed in many ways, including:

• being honest and saying what you think without being aggressive or overly critical
• openly giving support to colleagues
• sharing information
• listening to advice given
• helping everybody feel valued for their contribution to the team.

It is important that you try to do something about the things you find stressful. A particularly difficult area is if you witness **bad practice**, such as the maltreatment of a patient (including verbal abuse). It is important to discuss this with the staff member concerned, and report it to the person immediately senior to you. Physical abuse *must* be reported to the person in charge immediately. If you fail to do so not only will you feel stressed, but you will be collaborating by failing to report the incident and allowing someone to continue to carry out bad practice.

Stress and clients/residents

Studies have shown that people in care often feel very stressed. It is easy to see why if we think about a person who is about to enter a nursing home, for example.

One of the main reasons is their feeling of uncertainty about what is going to happen next. Because we are familiar with our work environment we sometimes forget that to our residents the care setting is a strange and disturbing place.

Accounts by patients in hospital show that lack of communication is a major theme. As a care assistant you may have far more conversation with the patient than senior staff, and are therefore in a unique position to put patients at ease. On admission to residential care, if the patient can go with you, show them the layout of the home, explain the routine and how to recognise the different types of staff.

A very interesting development in recent years has been the introduction of complementary therapies. Massage and aromatherapy have been found especially useful in relieving people's stress, and they may be useful in your care setting.

Women and stress

The majority of care assistants are women, who as a group may have extra stress not experienced by male colleagues.

Child care

Women with children may have particular practical difficulties, such as fitting in work hours around their children. Problems can also arise because of the economic necessity of working, while feeling guilty about leaving children in the care of other people. Financial pressures may also be evident because of the high cost of childminders and nursery placements.

There are no easy solutions. It is important that when you experience problems you discuss them – possibly with your manager. Many are sympathetic and have had similar problems themselves. Employers are becoming more enlightened, and some offer workplace creches and job share schemes.

Sexual harassment

Another recently identified cause of workplace stress, predominantly experienced by women, is sexual harassment – unwanted physical contact, offensive flirtations, constantly being asked out, unwelcome, sexist and patronising language, and sexual assault.

Dealing with these situations is difficult. If harassment occurs it should be reported to a senior person immediately. You may wish to seek advice from others – possibly from your union representative.

Points to remember

1. Stress is a response to threat.
2. It is generally recognised that caring for people with dementia is stressful.
3. Key life events are known to be stressful.
4. You will have physical symptoms if you are experiencing stress.
5. An important way to deal with stress is to talk to someone you can trust.
6. Try to identify stressful parts of your life, and if possible remove the cause or seek ways to deal with the problem.
7. Poor communication is a major cause of stress to people with dementia.
8. If bad practice is witnessed it must be reported to a senior person.
9. Sexual harassment should not be tolerated in the workplace.
10. Stress can be a beneficial experience if successfully overcome.

Glossary of terms

Abuse. Physical, verbal or emotional mistreatment or exploitation of another person against their best interests.

Accreditation of Prior Learning (for NVQ). Assessment of an individual's past achievements against national standards.

Acute. Used to describe an illness or condition that is of relatively short duration, and usually severe.

Advocate. A person who supports, encourages, defends and negotiates on behalf of another by representing them where they are unsure or unable to represent themselves.

AIDS (Acquired Immunodeficiency Syndrome – see also HIV). A condition caused by a virus called Human Immunodeficiency Virus (HIV). It damages the defence system so that the body cannot fight infection. It is passed on via body fluids such as blood, semen and vaginal fluids.

Allergy. A reaction to a substance to which a person is sensitive, eg fur, dust, alcohol, certain foods, insect stings and medicines. Usually causes skin rashes, but can be more severe causing difficulty with breathing due to swelling of the throat and airway. Death can occur. (See also Anaphylaxis).

Alzheimer's disease (see also Dementia). A form of dementia characterised by changes to the brain, although the particular cause is unknown. Loss of memory and intellectual function, disorientation, apathy and difficulty with coordinating movement, speech and thoughts, are common features.

Amnesia. Loss of memory.

Anaemia. Shortage of the oxygen-carrying part (haemoglobin) of the blood's red cells. This may be because the body is losing too much haemoglobin (eg due to bleeding) or because it is not making enough (eg due to a shortage of iron in the diet).

Anaesthetic. A substance that can cause temporary loss of the sensation of pain or consciousness. As a "local" anaesthetic it numbs a specific part of the body only. As a "general" anaesthetic it causes the patient to lose consciousness.

Analgesics. Medicines that provide relief from pain.

Anaphylactic shock. Severe reaction causing swelling of the airway and possible respiratory and cardiac arrest. It can occur when a medicine or injection is given; throughallergy or being bitten or stung by an insect.

Angina. Chest pain due to oxygen shortage in the heart muscles. Caused by narrowing or blockage of the coronary arteries which supply the heart muscle with oxygen.

Antibiotics. Medicines which either kill bacteria or stop them multiplying. They have no effect on a virus.

Anticonvulsant drugs. Medicines used to treat epilepsy.

Anti-depressant drugs. Medicines that are used in the treatment of depression. These drugs act upon and stimulate parts of the nervous system.

Anti-emetics. Medicines used to prevent nausea and sickness.

Anti-histamine. Medicines and creams used to counter symptoms of allergic reaction, eg irritation and itching of the skin.

Anus (see also Colon and Rectum). The muscular ring at the end of the intestinal canal.

Anxiety state. A condition in which the individual is so worried about a certain situation, that their life is severely restricted. The main characteristic is the inability to relax.

Arteriosclerosis. A gradual loss of elasticity in the walls of arteries due to thickening and the build up of calcium and cholesterol deposits. This may cause decreased blood flow and oxygen supply to essential parts of the brain and body.

Artery. A blood vessel carrying blood containing oxygen around the body.

Arthritis (see also Osteoarthritis and Rheumatoid Arthritis). Inflammation causing pain, stiffness or swelling in one or more joints.

Aseptic. Free from germs and bacteria that cause infection.

Assessment. The systematic collection of information by observing, interviewing and examining an individual and their social environment in order to develop a plan of care.

Assessment (for NVQ). The process of collecting evidence and making judgements on whether national standards have been met.

Assessors (for NVQ). Individuals approved by assessment centres to judge evidence of competence.

Asthma. A condition in which the tubes of the lung have a fluctuating and reversible tendency to narrow causing breathlessness, coughing, wheezing or chest tightness. It may be triggered by an allergy.

Audiometer. Machine used to test hearing.

Autopsy. See post mortem.

Awards in care. A set of NVQs at Level 2 and 3 with wide availability across health and social care.

Barrier cream. A cream, usually water based, that is applied to the skin to prevent drying or damage where for example a person may be incontinent.

Benign. When describing a tumour, means favourable, non-cancerous, usually contained within a capsule and not spreading to other parts of the body.

Bereavement. The human response to loss, usually as a result of a person dying. It also occurs when a person has lost something personal and important to them, such as their home, or a limb.

Blood pressure. The force of blood in the arteries measured in millimetres of mercury by a machine called a sphygmomanometer. Blood pressures are written down as two figures. The top figure is called "systolic" and the bottom figure is called "diastolic".

Bradycardia. A marked slowing of the rate of the heart.

Braille. A system of writing and printing by means of raised points representing letters which allows blind and partially sighted people to read by touch.

Bronchitis. Inflammation of the air tubes of the lungs. It may be "acute" due to infection, or "chronic" due to excessive production of mucus caused by many factors including pollution and smoking.

Bronchodilators. Medicines used to widen the lung airways.

Cancer. A large group of diseases which are linked together. In each case there is uncontrolled new abnormal tissue growth of the affected part/s of the body. The outlook for each cancer sufferer depends on site and type of the growth.

Capillaries. Tiny blood vessels that lie between arteries bringing blood to the tissues, and veins taking blood away.

Cardiac arrest. Used to describe a situation in which the heart suddenly stops beating.

Cardio-pulmonary resuscitation (CPR). The technique used to try and restart a heart after a person has had a cardiac arrest. Includes breathing into the person's lungs and externally massaging the heart in a regular and systematic way.

Carer. The term usually applied to a person who provides care at home without receiving a salary or wage. Most often it is a female relative of a dependent person.

Cataract. A clouding of the lens of the eye preventing light passing through it. Vision becomes very dim or is lost.

Catheter. A tube which is passed into the body to drain away fluids. The most common is the urinary catheter for draining the bladder.

Cerebrovascular accident (CVA). See stroke.

Cervix. The neck of the womb.

Chemotherapy. Treatment of disease by medicines or chemicals. The term is often used for cancer treatment, which can make the person feel very unwell and cause hair loss.

Chronic. A term used to describe a long-standing and continued disease process. There may be progressive deterioration (sometimes despite treatment).

Cognition. Consciously knowing, understanding and having insight into personal and environmental events. The person may not necessarily be able to take action.

Colic. A sharp pain resulting from spasm of a muscle, commonly the stomach and gut.

Colon (see also Anus and Rectum). A part of the large intestine that absorbs nutrients and fluid from the diet. It ends at the anus.

Colostomy. See Stoma.

Competence (for NVQ). The ability to perform an activity to the agreed standard. The assessment of competence forms the basis for NVQs and SVQs.

Compress. Soft pad of gauze or cloth used to apply heat, cold or medications to the surface of the body.

Concussion. A temporary loss of consciousness due to a knock on the head. The person becomes pale, has a feeble pulse and shallow breathing.

Confusion. Condition in which consciousness is clouded, so that the individual is unable to think clearly or act rationally. Confusional states may be temporary, due to acute illness (toxic confusional states), or long term and irreversible.

Constipation. Incomplete or infrequent action of the bowels, due to lack of muscle activity, insufficient fluids or inadequate diet.

Continence (see also Incontinence). The ability to control the functions of passing urine or faeces when desired.

Contra-indication. A reason for not doing something, such as giving a medicine as this could have an adverse effect.

Coronary artery disease. Narrowing or blockage of the arteries supplying the heart with oxygen. Usually due to blockage of the coronary arteries. Also known as coronary heart disease or coronary vascular disease.

Counselling. A skilled method of listening to and talking with a person or a group of people, to enable them to overcome a problem, make a decision or accept circumstances.

Culture. The values, attitudes, lifestyle and customs shared by a group of people, passed from one generation to the next.

Cyanosed. Bluish discolouration of the skin, particularly the lips, due to shortage of oxygen supply.

Cytology. The microscopic study of the cells of the body.

Defaecation. The act of opening the bowels.

Dehydration. Excessive loss of fluid from the body caused by vomiting, diarrhoea or sweating, or inadequate fluid intake.

Dementia (see also Alzheimer's disease). An organic mental illness caused by changes to the brain. This may be a result of disease or damage. The principal changes include inability to learn and retain information, inability to recall recent events, and feelings of anxiety and depression. This can lead to disorientation and confused behaviour.

Depression. A profound sadness, distinct from normal bereavement or loss. Its features include reduced enjoyment, slowness and a lack of interest in life or the lives of others.

Dexterity. The ability to use fingers and hands to undertake everyday activities.

Diabetes. Failure of the pancreas in the body to produce insulin, or failure of the body to use the insulin correctly. Insulin breaks down sugary foods, allowing the body to use it for energy. Diabetes results in too much sugar circulating in the blood. Normal body functioning, eg wound healing, is affected. It may be treated by diet alone, medicines or insulin.

Digoxin. One of the earliest discovered medicines which was found to have a beneficial effect on the failing heart.

Disorientation. A state of confusion in which an individual has lost a sense of where they are, what time it is and/or what they are doing.

Diuretic. A medicine which stimulates the kidney to produce more urine.

Diverticulitis. A condition in which there is inflammation of small pockets (diverticulae) of large bowel which stick through the muscle surrounding the bowel at weak points. Generally caused by long-standing constipation.

Down's syndrome. A congenital disorder caused by an extra chromosome. The person may have marked learning difficulties and heart problems.

Dysarthria. A speech disorder caused by poor muscle movement or poor muscle co-ordination, often following a stroke.

Dyslexia. Difficulty with reading and writing.

Dysphagia. Difficulty with swallowing.

Dysphasia. Language disorder which may affect understanding, speaking, reading and writing (often due to a stroke).

Eczema. A condition of the skin causing dryness, flaking and extreme itching.

Elimination. The removal of waste matter from the body.

Encephalitis. Inflammation of the brain, usually due to a virus.

Enema. Procedure involving the introduction of a fluid into the rectum for cleansing or therapeutic purposes.

Enteral feeding. Provision of nutrients through a tube directly into the stomach when the person cannot chew or swallow food but can digest and absorb the nutrients.

Epilepsy. A condition in which excessive or unregulated electrical activity in the brain causes fits. These may involve the whole body with loss of consciousness ("grand mal") or parts of the body, involving perhaps a short loss of full consciousness, known as "petit mal" fits. "Focal fits" are said to occur when only one part of the body, eg arms or legs, is affected.

Ethnicity (see also Culture). A group's sense of identity associated with race, heritage, upbringing and values.

Evidence (for NVQ). Proof in support of the judgement made by an assessor that a candidate is competent.

Exertion. The amount of effort a person puts into carrying out a task. This may be physical, in walking or getting out of bed. It can also be mental, for example struggling to remember recent events.

Faeces. Waste matter which is indigestible (such as fibre) excreted by the bowel.

Fainting. A temporary loss of consciousness due to a fall in blood pressure. The person usually falls to the floor, as this is the way in which the body attempts to restore the blood circulation, so that oxygen can reach the brain.

Fatigue. State of extreme exhaustion or loss of strength.

Fibre (in diet). Used to describe food that is high in roughage, indigestible, and which stimulates the action of the intestine (bowel).

Flatulence. Excessive wind, usually causing discomfort/pain.

Fracture. A broken bone. Signs and symptoms include pain, swelling, loss of power and shortening of the affected limb.

Gangrene. Death of body tissue usually due to loss of blood supply.

Genital. Relates to the sexual organs of the man or woman.

Glaucoma. A condition in which abnormally high fluid pressure inside the eye can cause permanent damage.

Guarding. A defensive action that a person may take to safeguard themselves or to prevent any pain. It may include not wishing to talk about difficult subjects or holding oneself in a comfortable position that prevents physical pain.

Haemorrhoids. Piles.

Heart attack. Damage to an area of the heart muscle due to obstruction of the artery supplying this area with blood. Usually preceded by extreme chest pain.

Heart failure. The failure by the heart to pump blood around the body efficiently. The most common symptoms are breathlessness, tiredness and swollen ankles.

Hemiplegia. Paralysis of one side of the body. Usually caused by stroke or as a result of injury or disease to the brain.

Hernia. Protrusion of an organ from its normal position in the body into another. The most common is the inguinal hernia in which bowel pushes through defects in the muscle of the groin. Also known as a "rupture".

HIV (Human Immunodeficiency Virus). The family of viruses that causes AIDS.

Hydrocephalus. Accumulation of fluid in and around the brain.

Hypertension (see also Blood pressure). A condition in which the blood pressure is higher than it should be for an individual person.

Hypotension. A condition in which the blood pressure is lower than it should be.

Hypothermia. Body temperature below the usual value of 37 degrees centigrade. At about 35 degrees centigrade confusion and listlessness may begin. Below 33 degrees centigrade the breathing and pulse rate and blood pressure may start to fall. If prolonged, death may occur.

Ileostomy (see Stoma).

Impairment. Reduction or weakening of any body function.

Incontinence (see also Continence). The inability to control the passage of urine or faeces until a suitable time and place is found. Urinary incontinence may occur when abdominal pressure, through coughing or lifting heavy weights, causes urine to leak from the bladder and urethra. Faecal incontinence is caused by a loss of control of the anus. Disorientation may also cause incontinence.

Infarct. An area of the body which is damaged or dies as a result of not receiving enough oxygen from its arteries. This supply failure is usually due to a blockage or haemorrhage from the artery. Frequently used as "coronary" or "myocardial" infarct to describe the damage done to heart muscle after a heart attack.

Infusion. Introduction of a substance, such as a medicine in fluid form, directly into a vein or under the skin. May be attached to a mechanical pump to ensure that the correct amount is given over a period of time.

Insomnia. Difficulty getting to sleep or staying asleep.

Intestine. The bowel.

Intractable. Commonly used in reference to pain, that is difficult to control or cure.

Larynx. The voice organ. Vocal cords of elastic tissue are spread across it. The vibrations and contractions of these produce the changes in the pitch of the voice.

Laxative. A medicine to encourage passing faeces.

Malabsorption. The failure of the gut to absorb nutrients and food. It can lead to malnutrition.

Malignant. A type of tumour that spreads and grows uncontrollably.

Malnutrition (see also nutrition). Under-nourishment due to poor diet or disease that prevents absorption of essential nutrients.

Medication (see also Sedation and Tranquilliser). Used to describe tablets, liquids or injections used with the aim of improving a person's physical or mental condition.

Melaena. The production of black, tarry stools containing blood from the upper part of the gut.

Metabolism. The sum total of the chemical processes that occur in living organisms, resulting in growth, production of energy, elimination of waste material.

Micturition. The act of emptying the bladder of urine.

Motor neurone disease. A disease in which there is progressive destruction of some of the nerves responsible for stimulating muscles. This causes weakness and problems with movement, breathing and swallowing; the cause is unknown.

Motor strength. The strength of the muscle which stimulates the limbs and body to move.

Mucous membrane. A mucus-secreting membrane that lines body cavities (eg lungs) or passages that are open to the external environment (eg mouth, nose, vagina).

Mucus. The protective secretion of the mucus membranes.

Multiple sclerosis. An often fluctuating, sometimes progressive disease of the brain and spinal cord in which plaques replace normal nerve tissue. This can cause a range of symptoms, including difficulty with coordinating movement, incontinence and problems with vision and speech.

Muscular dystrophy. A group of muscle disorders which are usually passed on through families and become apparent in childhood and adolescence.

National Council for Vocational Qualifications (NCVQ). Sets out the structure and framework of vocational qualifications for England, Wales and Northern Ireland. (SCOTVEC is the equivalent for Scotland.)

Nausea. The sensation of feeling sick.

Nebuliser. Equipment that adds drops of water or medicine to compressed air or oxygen so that it can be absorbed more effectively or dislodge mucus in the air passages and lungs.

Neurological. Relating to the body's brain and nerves.

Neuro-transmitters. Chemical substances that help to pass a signal down a nerve.

Nutrition. The intake of nutrients (in food and drink) and their assimilation into body tissue.

NVQs – National Vocational Qualifications. Practical work-based qualifications for care assistants.

Oedema. Excess tissue fluid, often around ankles, at the base of the spine or in the heart and lungs.

Osteoarthritis. A form of arthritis occurring in the joints of older people. It is usually very painful. There is destruction of the spongy pads between bones, and small bony growths at the edges of the bone joint.

Palliative. Treatment that relieves or reduces uncomfortable symptoms, such as pain, but does not provide a cure.

Paralysis. Loss of movement (but not sensation) in a muscle or group of muscles normally under the person's control. May be due to damage to the muscle itself or its nerve supply.

Parkinsonism. Symptoms such as shaking or trembling, rhythmical muscular tremors, rigidity and a mask-like face that shows no emotion. Thumb and fore fingers may move in a "rolling" fashion. It can be caused by tranquillisers.

Peak flow. The measurement of air as it is expelled from the lungs.

Performance criteria (for NVQ). A set of outcomes related to an element of performance by which an assessor can judge that a candidate can work to the required standard.

Personality. The mental make-up of a person. The way that they respond is influenced by life events and experiences, and their attitudes to situations.

Photophobia. Intolerance to light.

Pneumonia. Inflammation of the lungs due to bacterial, viral or fungal infections.

Prescription. A legal document that must be used and signed by a doctor for issuing medicines. It must contain the name, dose and frequency of the medicines.

Pressure sore. An area of skin and underlying tissues which dies as a result of pressure persistently preventing the flow of blood through its blood vessels. It can cause an ulcer or sore to develop, particularly if the skin is broken.

Prognosis. The outlook for a person with a disease, in terms of disability and death.

Prostate. A gland at the base of the bladder in men. It may become enlarged due to disease or old age, causing difficulty in passing urine.

Prosthesis. Manufactured substitute for a part of the body (for example an artificial leg, false teeth, breast).

Pruritus. Itching.

Pulse. The regular expansion and contraction of an artery produced by waves of pressure as blood is pumped through.

Pyrexia. Raised body temperature.

Quality Assurance (see also Audit and Standard). A system of evaluating and auditing the standards of a service to ensure that the best possible service is provided in terms of value for money and client satisfaction.

Racism. Discrimination against a person on the grounds of skin colour and/or ethnic origin.

Range statements (for NVQ). The breadth of contexts in which a candidate is expected to demonstrate competence (linked to an element of competence).

Recovery position. The safest position in which to place a person who is unconscious.

Rectum (see also Colon). The lower end of the bowel leading out to the anus.

Rehabilitation. The process by which a team of workers restores a person who has had a serious illness or injury to as near as possible their previous state of health.

Reminiscence therapy. Active participation by individuals or groups, using past life events to understand the reasons for their mental health problems. The past can also be used as a basis to share concerns and anxieties, since people with dementia are more likely to have a better memory for long term events than for more recent events.

Respiratory arrest. Used to describe a situation in which a person stops breathing, but before the heart stops beating. There can be more than one cause.

Respite. Temporary relief services for the main carer of a dependent person in the home or other setting.

Rheumatism. The term is loosely applied to any pain of unknown cause in joints or muscles. Small swellings may appear under the skin, particularly around bony ridges. There may be fever, sweating and pain and joint stiffness.

Rheumatoid arthritis. Arthritis occurring in the small and large joints of people of all ages. The cause is unknown.

Role reversal. A situation in which a person exchanges a pattern of behaviour with another. For example a daughter may have to take on a mothering role to her own mother if she requires care.

Sacrum. Part of the lower end of the spine.

Sedative (see also Medication and Tranquilliser). Having a calming or soothing effect.

Sexuality. A part of the human personality that relates in physical, emotional and social dimensions to the way a person identifies and values themself. It includes their gender, appearance and sexual preferences.

Sharps. Any piece of equipment used that could cause injury by stabbing or cutting a person if not disposed of safely.

Shock. This may arise out of fear or pain, it may also be the result of loss of blood, a reaction to medicines, or contact with electrical currents. It is the condition in which there is a sudden fall in blood pressure, which if untreated will lead to a lack of oxygen in the tissues.

Sphincter. A muscular ring which surrounds the opening of a hollow organ, such as the bladder. It controls the escape of the content of the organ until a suitable time.

Sprain. An injury to a ligament when the joint it is supporting is forced through a range of movements greater than normal, without dislocation or fracture.

Sputum. Excess secretion from the lungs that contains mucus and saliva. It may also contain bacteria.

Standard. A guide that serves as a basis for measuring how good or bad a particular service or practice is. (See also Audit and Quality Assurance.)

Stereotype. A commonly held belief about a behaviour, individual or group that is not always true.

Stethoscope. A device for listening to sounds within the body, such as heart beat, bowel sounds and breathing, that cannot otherwise be heard by the human ear.

Stoma. A surgical procedure in which an opening is made on the abdominal wall to allow the passage of intestinal contents (colostomy and ileostomy) or urine (urostomy) from the bladder.

Stool. Formed faeces passed from the bowel..

Stress. Stress reactions, both physical and mental, occur when the individual is unable to cope with all the demands made upon them. If extreme, it may be called "burn-out".

Stroke (see also Cerebrovascular accident). A rapid brain disorder usually caused by a blockage in or haemorrhage from one of the main arteries of the brain. Speech and movement are commonly affected. Other functions may be damaged depending upon which artery is affected. Recovery depends on the extent of the damage.

Subcutaneous. Relates to an injection or infusion given into the skin tissue at a 45 degree angle, rather than into the muscle (intramuscular).

Syringe driver. A battery-driven device for giving drugs (usually pain killers) over a period of time via a subcutaneous needle under the skin.

Systole. The maximum level of blood pressure measured between heart contractions.

Tachycardia. A marked increase in the rate of the heart.

Thrombosis. The formation of a blood clot on the lining of an artery or vein which may partially or completely block the blood flow through it.

Thrush. A fungal infection usually affecting the mucous membranes such as the mouth and vagina.

Toxin. Any poisonous compound. It may be caused by bacteria multiplying in the body.

Tracheostomy. A temporary or permanent surgical opening above the Adam's apple. It allows a person to breathe when the throat or upper airway is diseased or damaged.

Tranquilliser (see also Medication and Sedation). Medicines that allay anxiety and have a calming effect on the person. They may also prevent them from feeling pain.

Trauma. A wound or injury, physical or emotional. Emotional trauma can be a cause of mental illness.

Tumour. A lump or swelling in the body that is not inflamed. A benign tumour does not grow in other parts of the body. A malignant tumour may spread to other organs.

Ulcer. An erosion and inflammation of the skin or mucous membranes. Examples include venous leg ulcers, caused by poor skin condition and poor return of blood to the heart. Arterial leg ulcers are caused by poor blood supply.

Universal precautions. The wearing of gloves and protective clothing, and correct cleaning and disposal of waste, to prevent the spread of infection from blood and body fluids.

Ureters. The tubes which drain urine from the kidneys into the bladder.

Urethra. The tube that carries urine from the bladder to outside the body.

Urine. Waste products in liquid form that are produced in the kidney and emptied from the body via the bladder.

Urinary tract infection. An infection that affects the bladder or the urethra. It may result in the person wanting to pass urine frequently, cause pain and a stinging sensation.

Urostomy See Stoma.

Varicose veins. A condition, usually of the lower leg, in which the veins are swollen and may be twisted due to structural changes in the walls or valves of the vessels. These veins have difficulty returning blood back to the heart. Knocks to varicose veins can cause painful leg ulcers in older people.

Vascular. Relating to blood vessels, usually arteries or veins.

Vein. A vessel carrying blood from the capillaries back to the heart after oxygen has been removed by the tissues and organs that need it.

Vertigo. A feeling of dizziness accompanied by a feeling that either oneself or one's surroundings are spinning.

Useful addresses

All organisations listed below welcome the inclusion of a stamped addressed envelope with your enquiry.

Action for Dysphasic Adults, Canterbury House, 1 Royal Street, London SE1 7LL. Tel: 020 7261 9572.

Action on Elder Abuse, Age Concern England, Astral House, 1268 London Road, London SW16 4ER. Helpline: 020 8679 8000.

Afro Caribbean Mental Health Association, 49 Effra Road, London SW2 1BZ. Tel: 020 7737 3603.

Age Concern England, Astral House, 1268 London Road, London SW16 4ER. Tel: 020 8679 8000.

Age Concern Cymru, 4th Floor, 1 Cathedral Road, Cardiff CF1 9SD. Tel: 029 2037 1566.

Age Concern Northern Ireland, 3 Lower Crescent, Belfast BT7 1NR. Tel: 028 9024 5729.

Age Concern Scotland, 113 Rose Street, Edinburgh EH2 3DT. Tel: 0131 220 3345.

Age Exchange Reminiscence Centre, 11 Blackheath Village, London SE3 9LA. Tel: 020 8318 9105.

Alzheimer Scotland – Action on Dementia, 22 Drumsheugh Gardens, Edinburgh EH3 7RN. Tel: 0131 243 1453.

Alzheimer's Society, Gordon House, 10 Greencoat Place, London SW1P 1PH. Tel: 020 7306 0606. Helpline: 0845 300 0336.

Alzheimer's Society Wales Development Office, Tonna Hospital, Tonna, Neath, Neath and Port Talbot SA11 3LX. Tel: 01639 633400.

Alzheimer's Society (Northern Ireland), 403 Lisburn Road, Belfast BT9 7EW. Tel: 028 9066 4100.

Association for Continence Advice, 102a Astra House, Arklow Road, London SE14 6EB. Tel: 020 8692 4680 www.aca.uk.com

British Complementary Medicine Association, PO Box 5122, Bournemouth BH8 0WG Tel: 0845 345 5977 Email: info@bcma.co.uk www.bcma.co.uk

British Dietetic Association, 5th floor, Charles House, 148/9 Great Charles Street, Queensway, Birmingham B3 3HT Tel: 0121 200 8080 info@bda.uk.com www.bda.uk.com

British Federation of Care Home Proprietors, 840 Melton Road, Thurmaston, Leicester LE4 8BN. Tel: 01162 640095.

British Red Cross Society, 9 Grosvenor Crescent, London SW1X 7EJ. Tel: 020 7235 5454. Volunteer beauty care and other services.

BTEC (Business and Technology Education Council), Central House, Upper Woburn Place, London WC1H 0HH. Tel: 020 7393 4494.

Carers National Association, Ruth Pitter House, 20-25 Glasshouse Yard, London EC1A 4JS. Tel: 020 7490 8818. Helpline: 0345 573369.

Carers National Association in Wales, Pantglas Industrial Estate, Bedwas, Newport, Gwent NP1 8DR. Tel: 02920 880176.

Carers National Association in Scotland, 3rd Floor, 162 Buchanan Street, Glasgow G1 2LL. Tel: 0141 333 9495.

Centre for Policy on Ageing, 25-31 Ironmonger Row, London EC1V 3QP. Tel: 020 7253 1787.

Chinese Mental Health Association, Oxford House, Derbyshire Street, London E2 6HG. Tel: 020 7613 1008.

Christian Council on Ageing, Mrs Margaret Young, New Cottage, The Square, Parwich, Derbyshire DE6 1QJ. Tel/fax: 01335 390484..

City and Guilds, 1 Giltspur Street, London EC1A 9DD. Tel: 020 7294 2468.

CNEOPSA (Care Needs of Ethnic Older Persons Suffering from Alzheimer's), PRIAE London, Boardman House, 64 Broadway, London E15 1NT Tel: 020 8432 0260 Email: hannah.zeilig@priae.org www.priae.org

Continence Foundation, 307 Hatton Square, 16 Baldwins Gardens, London EC1N 2PH. Tel: 020 7404 6875. Helpline: 020 7831 9831.

Counsel and Care, Twyman House, 16 Bonny Street, London NW1 9PG. Tel: 020 7485 1550. Helpline: 0845 300 7585.

Cruse – Bereavement Care, Cruse House, 126 Sheen Road, Richmond, Surrey TW9 1UR. Tel: 020 8940 4818.

Disabled Living Foundation, 380-384 Harrow Road, London W9 2HU. Tel: 020 7289 6111. Helpline: 0870 603 9177.

English National Board for Nursing, Midwifery and Health Visiting, Victory House, 170 Tottenham Court Road, London W1P 0HA. Tel: 020 7388 3131.

General Social Care Council, Goldings House, 2 Hay's Lane, London SE1 2HB Tel: 020 7397 5100 Email: info@gscc.org.uk; www.gscc.org.uk

Health and Safety Executive (HSE), Broad Lane, Sheffield, S3 7HQ. Tel: 0114 289 2500.

Health Education Authority, Trevelyan House, 30 Great Peter Street, London SWC1P 2HW. Tel: 020 7222 5300.

Help the Aged, 16-18 St James's Walk, Clerkenwell Green, London EC1R 0BE. Tel: 020 7253 0253.

Horticultural Therapy, Goulds Ground, Vallis Way, Frome, Somerset BA11 3DW. Tel: 01373 464782.

Huntington's Disease Association, 108 Battersea High Street, London SW11 3HP. Tel: 020 7223 9489.

Listening Books, 12 Lant Street, London SE11 1QH. Tel: 020 7407 9417. Postal audio library on standard cassette tape and on extended playing

Dementia Services Development Centres

Each of these centres is a resource for local information on best practice, training and resources for dementia care. Centres in other areas of the country are planned. Latest information from The Journal of Dementia Care (020 7720 2108 ext. 206).

SCOTLAND
Dementia Services
Development Centre
University of Stirling
Stirling FK9 4LA.
Tel: 01786 467740
Email: mtmarshall@stir.ac.uk
www.stir.ac.uk/dsdc

NORTH EAST
Dementia North
Allendale House
Northumbria University
Newcastle upon Tyne
NE7 7XA
Tel: 0191 215 6110
Email: hs.dementianorth@
unn.ac.uk
http://online.northumbria.
ac.uk/faculties/hswe/
research/Dementia.htm

NORTH WEST
North West Dementia Centre
Dover Street Building
University of Manchester
Manchester M13 9PL
Tel: 0161 275 5682
Email: nwdc.man.ac.uk
www.pssru.man.ac.uk

CENTRAL
Trent DSDC (being developed)
Trent Dementia Services
Development Centre
Professor James Lindesay,
Psychiatry for the Elderly,
Leicester General Hospital,
Gwendolen Road,
Leicester LE5 4PW
Tel: 0116 258 8161
Email: jebl1@le.ac.uk

Dementia Plus West Midlands
Warstones Resource Centre
Warstones Drive, Penn,
Wolverhampton WV4 4PG
Tel: 01902 575064
Email: dementiaplus.wm@
whc-tr.nhs.uk
www.wmpmh.org.uk/
dementiaplus

Oxford Dementia Centre
Institute of Public Care
Roosevelt Drive
Headington
Oxford OX3 7XR
Tel: 01865 761798
Email:
dementia@brookes.ac.uk
www.brookes.ac.uk

SOUTH EAST
London Centre for
Dementia Care
UCL, Wolfson Building
48 Riding House Street
London W1N 8AA
Tel/fax: 020 7679 9588
Email:
margot.lindsay@ucl.ac.uk
www.ucl.ac.uk/lcdc

**BRADFORD
DEMENTIA GROUP**
National resource for information, research, training (including Dementia Care Mapping) and publications.
Bradford Dementia Group
School for Health Studies
Bradford University
Unity Building
25 Trinity Road
Little Horton
Bradford BD5 0BB
Tel: 01274 233996
Fax: 01274 236395
email: L.J.Fox@bradford.ac.uk
www.bradford.ac.uk\acad\
health\bdg

Dementia Service
Development Centre
South East
Canterbury Christ Church
University College
Canterbury
Kent CT1 1QU
Tel: 01227 782702
Email:dsdcse@canterbury.ac.uk
http://dementiacentre.cant.
ac.uk

SOUTH WEST
Dementia Voice
Blackberry Hill Hospital
Manor Road
Fishponds, Bristol
BS16 2EW
Tel: 0117 975 4863
Fax: 0117 975 4819
Email: office@dementia-
voice.org.uk
www.dementia-voice.org.uk

WALES
DSDC Wales is based in both
Bangor and Cardiff
Details from:
Lesley Prenderghast
Information Officer
Dementia Services
Development Centre
Neuadd Ardudwy
University of Wales Bangor
Holyhead Road
Bangor, LL57 2PX
Tel: 01248 382092
Email: dsdc@bangor.ac.uk
www.bangor.ac.uk/dsdc

REPUBLIC OF IRELAND
Ireland DSDC
St James's Hospital,
St James's Street
Dublin 8
Tel: 00353 1 416 2035
Email: dsidc@stjames.ie
www.dementia.ie

tapes. Machines available for loan for people with limited manual dexterity.

MIND/National Association for Mental Health, Granta House, 15-19 Broadway, London E15 4BQ. Tel: 020 8519 2122. Helpline: 020 8522 1728

Multiple Sclerosis Society of Great Britain and Northern Ireland, 25 Effie Road, London SW6 1EE. Tel: 020 7610 7171.

National Care Homes Association, 3rd Floor, Martin House, 84-86 Gray's Inn Road, London WC1X 8BQ. Tel: 020 71 831 7090.

National Council for Vocational Qualifications, 29 Bolton Street, London W1 7PD. Tel: 020 7509 5555.

Nutrition Advisory Group for Elderly People (NAGE), c/o British Dietetic Association (see also).

Open College, Portland Tower, Portland Street, Manchester M1 3LD. Tel: 0161 245 3300.

Open University, Information Office, Department of Health and Social Welfare, Milton Keynes MK7 6AA. Tel: 01908 653743.

PAT Dogs (Pet Aided Therapy Scheme), Rocky Bank, 4 New Road, Ditton, Kent ME20 6AD. Tel: 01732 848499.

Registered Nursing Homes Association, Calthorp House, Hagley Road, Birmingham B16 8QY. Tel: 0121 454 2511.

Relatives Association, 5 Tavistock Place, London WC1H 9SN. Tel: 020 7916 6055.

Royal College of Nursing of the UK, 20 Cavendish Square, London W1M 0AB. Tel: 020 7409 3333.

Royal College of Speech and Language Therapists, 2 White Hart Yard, London SE1 1NX. Tel: 020 7378 1200.

Social Care Association, Thornton House, Hook Road, Surbiton, Surrey KT6 5AN. Tel: 020 8397 1411.

TFH, 76 Barracks Road, Sandy Lane Industrial Estate, Stourport-on-Severn, Worcestershire DY13 9QB. Tel: 01299 827820. Games, puzzles, pastimes for disabled/older people.

Therapet Visiting Scheme, Minaird House, Machrihanish, Campbelltown, Argyll PA28 6PZ. Tel: 01586 810314.

United Kingdom Central Council For Nursing, Midwifery and Health Visiting, 23 Portland Place, London W1N 3AF. Tel: 020 7637 7181.

VOICES (Voluntary Organisations Involved in Caring in the Elderly Sector), c/o The Association of Charity Officers, Beechwood House, Wyllotts Close, Potters Bar, Herts EN6 2HN. Tel: 01707 651777.

Index